A Nursing Guide to Adult Moderate Sedation

A.G Davis BSN, RN, CSRN

Copyright © 2013 A.G Davis
All rights reserved.
ISBN-13: 978-1481915977
ISBN-10: 1481915975

DEDICATION

To all nurses who share my specialty.
To my family, anything is possible.

CONTENTS

	Acknowledgments	i
1	The Fundamentals	1
2	Regulatory Bodies & Other Resources	5
3	Credentialing and Education	13
4	Pre-Procedure	21
5	Intra-Procedure	36
6	Post-Procedure	58
7	Medications	66
8	Special Populations	108

Pediatrics & Geriatrics
Pregnancy and Lactation
Bariatric
Sleep Apnea
Chronic Obstructive & Pulmonary disease
Substance and Alcohol Abuse

9	Challenging Circumstances	150
10	Future Trends and Possibilities	166
	Appendix	176

ACKNOWLEDGMENTS

I want to start off by acknowledging the first person who inspired me, Dr. Stephen Bader. He motivated me to be more active in moderate sedation education. I want to thank, Ron Eslinger for being resourceful, inspirational, and serving your country.

To all my Interventional Radiology & Radiology colleagues for encouraging me to start a journey in moderate sedation education, policies, protocols, and standardization.

To those who peer interviewed this book, Sally Leonard, Chris Szymoniak, and Heather Malcolm, I appreciate your time and recommendations.

To Sally Leonard again for being my Jiminy Cricket.

To Jordan Maze, I thank you for your expertise and time in editing this book. You had by far the toughest job.

To my parents, thank you for creating such a stubborn child and giving inspirational words like "you got to want it" and "you can do anything".

Lastly, I want to thank my husband for always challenging and tolerating me.

Chapter 1

The Fundamentals

Sedation was once called general anesthesia or sedation. However, things started to change when dentistry started to use registered nurses in the 1980's to administer benzodiazepine with an opioid to healthy patients under the supervision of a dentist. Their intent was to provide decreased anxiety, pain and discomfort associated with medical procedures. The reason for the move from anesthesia services providing sedation to physician-nurse teams was as simple as supply vs. demand; there were more patients requiring sedation than individuals providing the sedation.

With the changes that occurred there came about the question of who was technically qualified to administer sedation. Nurses turned to their state board for answers, but because the concept of physician-nurse teams administrating sedation was newly developed there weren't clear guidelines to follow. Hence, our profession was born and with few practice guidelines, standards, or education and training.

In reality, it wasn't until 2002, when the American Society of Anesthesiologists (ASA)- an educational, research, and scientific association- developed a task force for non-anesthesiologists who administer sedation and analgesia (moderate & deep sedation). It was this task force which developed some practice guidelines and defined sedation/anesthesia into four levels, which have been endorsed by regulatory bodies, such as Center of Medicaid and Medicare (CMS) and the Joint Commission (TJC).

The Continuum and Definitions of Sedation

Approved by the ASA House of Delegates on October 27, 2004, and amended on October 21, 2009

Minimal Sedation (anxiolysis)

A drug-induced state during which patients respond normally to verbal commands. Although cognitive function and coordination may be impaired, ventilatory and cardiovascular functions are unaffected [1].

The following signs can be used to identify minimal sedation (anxiolysis):

- Normal response to verbal stimulation
- Airway unaffected
- Spontaneous ventilation unaffected
- Cardiovascular function unaffected

Moderate Sedation/Analgesia

Moderate sedation is a drug-induced depression of consciousness during which patients respond purposefully to verbal commands, either alone or accompanied by light tactile stimulation. No interventions are required to maintain a patent airway, and spontaneous ventilation is adequate [1].

This means the goal of Moderate Sedation is to:

- Decrease anxiety, pain, discomfort
- Promote amnesia for the patient
- Maintain cardiovascular functions
- Maintain adequate ventilation, homeostasis and circulation
- Maintain appropriate level of consciousness
- Ensure patient safety by recognizing potential for adverse complications

Deep Sedation/Analgesia

Deep sedation is a drug-induced depression of consciousness during which patients cannot be easily aroused but respond purposefully following repeated or painful stimulation. The ability to independently maintain ventilatory function may be impaired. Patients may require assistance in maintaining a patent airway, and spontaneous ventilation may be inadequate. Cardiovascular function is usually maintained [1].

The following signs highlight this depth of anesthesia:

- Purposeful response following repeated or painful stimulation
- Airway intervention may be required
- Spontaneous ventilation may be inadequate
- Cardiovascular function usually maintained

General Anesthesia

General anesthesia is a drug-induced loss of consciousness during which patients are not arousable, even by painful stimulation. The ability to independently maintain ventilatory function is often impaired [1].

- Patients often require assistance in maintaining a patent airway, and positive pressure ventilation may be required because of depressed spontaneous ventilation or drug-induced depression of neuromuscular function.

- Cardiovascular function may be impaired. General anesthesia will be performed by credentialed anesthesia providers under the standards of anesthesia care.

Why the sedation continuum is important?

It is important to understand the continuum of sedation because the response of any one patient may be unpredictable. For instance, a Licensed Independent Physician (LIP) with privileges may plan to moderately sedate a patient; however it doesn't mean that the patient will stay within the moderate sedation realm. Moderate sedation does not usually put a patient's breathing or heart function at risk, but a moderately sedated patient may progress to deep sedation. A patient can go from minimal to moderate to deep and then moderate again several times through out a case. The ASA recognizes this rationale and has developed practice guidelines that state moderate sedation must be monitored just as vigilantly as deep sedation and anesthesia. The ASA, CMS, and TJC also require that the practitioner (nurse & Physician) responsible *should* be capable of managing and rescuing a patient one level deeper than their intended plan. Hence the development of credentialing and privileging was created [1] [3].

Reference:

1. American Society Of Anesthesiology. (n.d.). *Continuum of depth of sedation:*. Retrieved from http://www.asahq.org/For-Healthcare-Professionals/Standards-Guidelines-and-Statements.aspx
2. Eslinger, R. (n.d.). *Moderate sedation policy & procedure*. Retrieved from http://sedationcertification.com/

3. Urman, R. D, & Kaye, A. D. (2012). *Moderate and deep sedation in clinical practice*. New York: Cambridge University Pres

Chapter 2

Regulatory Bodies & Other Resources:

Understanding Their Roles

Within the moderate sedation specialty, there are several reviewing regulatory bodies and nationally recognized organizations that play an important part in the practice of administrating Adult Moderate Sedation. For minimal, moderate, deep and general sedation administration, the federal and state regulatory bodies dictate regulations and develop guidelines. Accreditation bodies like The Joint Commission (TJC), enforce government regulations. Nationally recognized organizations like the ASA provide expert opinion, evidence based practice, and positions on the appropriate practices in the administration of sedation.

Federal

There is little regulation in regards to nurses and their scope of practice in administering moderate sedation. What is mentioned comes from The Center of Medicare and Medicaid Services and its relationship to institutions that participate in their services. So in other words if an institution participates with Medicare and Medicaid, then that institution has to follow specific standards and practice guidelines regulated by CMS in order to provide moderate sedation services by physician-nurse teams.

The Center of Medicare and Medicaid Services

In CMS Manual, 482.52 Condition of Participation: (Anesthesia Services) It states that "if the hospital furnishes anesthesia services, they must be provided in a well organized manner under the direction of a qualified doctor..." it further states that "the service is responsible for all anesthesia administered in the hospital". In other words the anesthesia department governs sedation through out the hospital, whether it is moderate, deep or general, and in any department (Radiology, Emergency room, Cath lab, Endo etc) within the hospital [1].

Anesthesia governing body, according to CMS:

- has to develop policies & procedures based on nationally recognized guidelines (482.12).
- determine the privileges to be granted to individual practitioners (482.22).
  - CMS only allows anesthesia professionals or other qualified non-anesthesiologist under state law to administer deep sedation. Mid-level practitioners and registered nurses are not permitted to administer deep sedation.
- establish qualifications and provisions of nurses who care for patients (482.22) and physicians who administer anesthesia (482.23).
- periodically review policies & procedures, adverse events, medication errors and other quality/safety indicators (482.21)

Furthermore, CMS (482.52) defines the levels of sedation and its continuum in accordance with the ASA guidelines. They also state that "rescue capacity is required as an essential component of anesthesia services, but also consistent with the requirements under the Patients Rights standard at 482.13". Meaning not only do they hold the ASA's sedation definitions as a gold standard, but they agree with the ASA in that institutions must have a system in place to rescue patients whose level of sedation becomes deeper than intended. CMS does give the organization "**freedom**" to define how it will determine that the individuals are able to perform the required types of rescue [1].

State

The state that one practices in may or may not address regulations with regards to scope of practice issues for registered nurses who administer moderate sedation. The state of West Virginia for example, doesn't mention anything about moderate sedation. This regulatory body only makes the statement, that as a registered nurse; I can not administer specific medications unless there under certain circumstances (see box 1).

Box 1

WV Board of Examiners for Registered Professional Nurses

Chp. 30, Article 7, Section 15

Oct 22, 2010

> It is not within the scope of practice for a professional registered nurse to administer anesthetics such as Ketamine, propofol, etomidate, sodium thiopental, methohexital, nitrous oxide and paralytics, except under the following circumstances:
>
>> Managing a continuous infusion of an anesthetic agent or paralytic for a patient who is intubated and ventilated in the acute care setting. Dose titration and bolus of agents to be administer to the intubated and ventilated patient may be implemented by RN's, based upon specific orders or protocols signed by qualified licensed physicians.
>>
>> Rapid Sequence Intubation- agents may be administered in the presence of a physician or advanced practiced registered nurse credentialed in emergency airway management and cardio vascular support.
>>
>> Chapter 30, article 7, section 15 for further explanation [9]

To find your state board of nursing regulation on sedation practices you can try going to this website http://sedationcertification.com/resources/position-statements/clickable-map/ created by Healthy Visions, a company that specializes in certifying health care providers in moderate sedation [6].

Policy & Procedures

Your institution, whether they participate with CMS or not, should have some sort of policy & procedure on sedation and the nurses role in this practice. There should be a statement on who can administer moderate sedation and what type of training is required, especially if the hospital is accredited by an agency such as Joint Commission (aka JCT), Health Facilities accreditation Program (HFAP), or Def Norske Veritas Healthcare, Inc (DNV) (the top three accrediting bodies for CMS).

Sedation policies and procedures according to CMS are to be developed by the department of anesthesiology. However, it is more beneficial to utilize a multidisciplinary team, involving anesthesia, nurses, and physicians with privileges to administer moderate sedation. A multidisciplinary team can help ensure continuity, addressing every department with in the institution that provides moderate sedation and any concerns that each provider may have. Institutional policies and procedures should encompass publicized recommended practice guidelines and position statements by professional organizations [2]. Adherence to state statutory law must also be incorporated into the policies and procedures. These aspects promote positive patient outcomes by having an integrated healthcare system that allows staff to be on the same page.

To find out whether one can administer moderate sedation under a privileged physician in your institution, see your establishment's policy & procedure on sedation. If one is unable to find any policy and procedures regarding moderate sedation and your role in it, try climbing the chain of command ladder. Promote the need for developing a policy and procedure for one's institution if there isn't one. The sole purpose of policies and procedures is to serve the organization, protect employees and provide consistent safe patient care.

Accreditation Agencies

Why do institutions use accrediting agencies and what role do they play in sedation?

Healthcare organizations don't have to use accreditation agencies however if an institution participates with CMS, then they need to. Although healthcare organizations can have CMS audit their performance in following CMS standards, CMS simply doesn't have the resources to audit healthcare organizations themselves [8]. When CMS can't audit all the institutions wanting to be certified and recertified in a timely manner, health care organizations can't participate in CMS services. When this occurs, healthcare establishments are unable to service CMS clients. Although CMS clients only represent 22% of those insured in the U.S., they use their CMS insurance more frequently than the average person.

The end result is limited amount of money comes into the institution. Relatively this means a lack of developing new technology and quality care to their facilities and region. So most healthcare organizations participate in CMS and in doing so they must be audited and certified through accredited agencies like TJC.

TJC is currently the leading accreditation agency in their industry. With the goal of helping hospitals become highly reliable organizations for developing safe effective care, TJC act as an auditor for CMS in over 15,000 healthcare organizations. They have aligned their standards in accordance to CMS's conditions of participation. Although they share many of the same standards between the two, TJC has developed several standards that are a little more in detail than CMS's. This is to ensure that patient safety is the number one priority for healthcare providers in the world of sedation administration [3].

In the next following chapters TJC's requirements for sedation and analgesia will be referred to. Especially topics like credentialing, privileging, monitoring, medication administration, phases of patient care and practice evaluation. As promised you will also be informed of the adult moderate sedation nurse's role within these standards.

Non Legal Organizations

Non Legal Organizations are nationally recognized societies or associations that have constructed position statements and/or practice guidelines. Here are some organizations that have made statements and practice guidelines that pertain to sedation and analgesia.

- American Academy of Pediatrics (AAP)
- American Association of Nurse anesthetists (AANA)
- American College of Cardiology (ACC),
- American College of Emergency Physicians (ACEP)
- American College of Radiology (ACR)
- Society of Interventional Radiology (SIR)
- Association for Radiologic & Imaging Nursing (ARIN)
- American Association of Moderate Sedation Nurses (AAMSN) *
- American Society for Gastrointestinal Endoscopy (ASGE) *
- American Society of Anesthesiologists (ASA) *
- Association of PeriOperative Registered Nurses (AORN)
- University Health-System Consortium (UHC)

*= favorites of the author

Institutional policies should be in accordance with position statements, clinical practice guidelines from nationally recognized organizations and state laws (box 2).

Why are these organizations position statements and practice guidelines so important? How do you know which organization position statements or practice guidelines to use if they are different?

Legally speaking, position statements and practice guidelines are a set of recommendations for patient care that recognizes a specific or assortment of approaches that a reasonable qualified health care provider would perform. Both can be incorporated into a policy but position statements are not based on clinical evidence. They are made from an expert panel based on opinion [7]. Practice guidelines are developed to help health care providers make clinical decisions from day to day [5]. Some practice guidelines are still based on tradition or authority, but recently more and more practice guidelines are becoming based on an examination of current evidence. CMS and health care providers are finding that sound foundation of evidence of what works best to achieve the greatest quality of care is essential [4].

Summary

Each regulatory body plays and important role in the administration and management of sedation and analgesia. If your institution participates with Medicare and Medicaid, then CMS sets the basic requirements for safe patient care. TJC evaluates your institutions performance in adhering to CMS requirements. State boards should provide nurses and physicians with a scope of practice addressing the administration and management of sedation, however not all do. Next your institution, regardless of CMS participation should have a policy on patient sedation. Any institutions that do participate in CMS must have a policy developed from anesthesia governing body [1]. Lastly, policies are behooved to incorporate requirements, standards and evidence based practice from regulatory bodies and non legal organizations.

Unfortunately, moderate sedation practice standards and guidelines don't come from one particular source. Throughout the United States (U.S) healthcare institutions have to piece together their policies and procedures based from federal and state regulations, accreditation bodies, and nationally recognized organizations. What can be provided in one state may not be able to be done in another state. What one nationally recognized organization recommends may not be the same as another well know organization. There is so much inconsistency throughout the country in this specialty that it leaves a lot of room for knowledge deficit and poor patient care. Hopefully in the future we will see a more organized system in place for the development and regulation of moderate sedation.

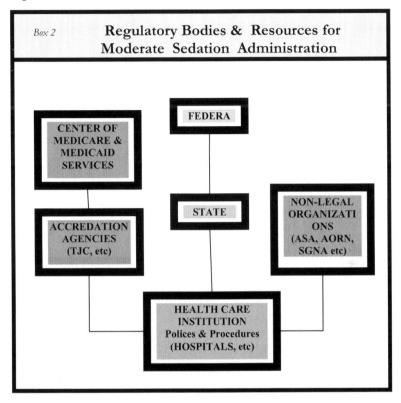

References:

1. Department of Health & Human Services, Centers for Medicare & Medicaid Services. (2011). *482.52 condition of participations: Anesthesia services* (100-07). Retrieved from website: http://www.cms.gov/Regulations-and-Guidance/Guidance/Manuals/Internet-Only-Manuals-IOMs-Items/CMS1201984.html

2. Kost, M. (2004). *Moderate sedation/analgesia.* (2nd ed.). St. Louis: Saunders.

3. Meldi, D., Rhoades, F. & Gippe, A. (2009, 01). *The big three: A side by side matrix comparing hospital accrediting agencies. Synergy*, 14-16. Retrieved from http://www.hfap.org/mediacenter/NAMSSSynergy JanFeb09_Accreditation_Grid.pdf

4. Phurrough, S. M. M. (n.d.). *Cms activities to advance evidence-based medicine*. Retrieved on 2013/01/09 from http://www.nhpf.org/library/handouts/Phurrough.slides_10-03-08.pdf

5. *Practice guidelines*. (n.d.). Retrieved on 2012/1/09 from http://medical-dictionary.thefreedictionary.com/practice guidelines

6. *Sedation certification*. (2012). Retrieved on 1/15/13, from http://sedationcertification.com/resources/position-statements/clickable-map/

7. Urman, R. D, & Kaye, A. D. (2012). *Moderate and deep sedation in clinical practice*. New York: Cambridge University Press.

8. Virginia Department of Health, Office of Licensure and Certification. (n.d.). *The accreditation option for deemed Medicare status*. Retrieved from website: http://www.vdh.state.vaus

9. *West Virginia board of examiners for registered professional nurses*. (n.d.). Retrieved on 1/15/13 from http://www.wvrnboard.com/

Chapter 3

Credentialing and Education

Knowing the minimum is all that is required but is that enough? In this chapter the credentialing and education process for adult moderate sedation privileging will be mentioned in detail.

The federal and state system in the U.S has the ultimate say in who is permitted to administer and manage moderate sedation to patients. Since the federal government has little regulation, then the state board (Medicine & Nurses) is the next regulatory body to address this position. The only problem is that not every state makes a statement on who can administer and manage a moderate sedation. If the state you reside in doesn't have a position on the practice, then your institution, especially if they participate with CMS and TJC are the next regulatory bodies to address this topic. CMS & TJC require health care institutions to implement a way to qualify a licensed independent practitioner to provide moderate sedation within their policies [1].

CMS states that:

- health care institutions must include criteria for determining privileges to be granted and a procedure for applying the criteria to requesting individuals (482.22) [1].
- intravenous medications administered by a healthcare person other than doctors of medicine or osteopathy, must have special training (482.23) [1].

CMS does not however state the type of specialized training an individual needs in order to become credentialed or privileged. In spite of this CMS and TJC does recognize that sedation is a continuum and it is not always able to predict how a patient will respond. Both organizations, therefore, deem a rescue capacity be in place, such as code or anesthesia team, in an institution. Each organization has the freedom to define how health care providers are able to perform rescue [1] [4]. TJC (PC.03.01) endorses CMS and further requires that those healthcare providers given permission to administer sedation have the ability to rescue one sedation level deeper than the intended level (nurse and physician) [5] [7].

So in other words, in order for an institution to be able to provide the service of moderate sedation by a nurse under the direct supervision of a physician:

1. There must be a rescue response team organized and in place prior to the service. An organization does however have the freedom to choose who the rescue team consist of.

   i. An example of this type of team may be a respiratory therapist, paramedic, nurse or anesthesiologist trained and privileged in airway rescue. Along with an airway rescue, your team may consist of an emergency department physician and a stat nurse.

2. The physician ordering the moderate sedation must be able to manage a patient one level deeper than the intended sedation level and so should the nurse.

   i. Physician should have Advanced Life Support (ACLS) or equivalent to be credentialed.

   ii. The nurse should also have the same type of training.

Having a rescue team is the minimal for a physician-nurse team to be credentialed. So for instance this means that according to TJC, CMS, and your state, an institution can hire a clinic nurse with no critical care training to administer moderate sedation under the supervision of a physician who may have never medically managed a patient. This doesn't seem to be the best quality of care that could be given to patient requiring moderate sedation.

Minimal training requirements are one of the biggest problems we as nurses face in the United States. There are simply no uniform guidelines, policies, protocols amongst organizations, provider groups, and even within the same organization. More importantly there isn't any specialized training for healthcare professionals to order and administer Adult Moderate Sedation, other than anesthesiology providers. The inability to reach a consensus on safe practice, appropriate training and guidelines threatens our ability as health care professionals to provide safe and consistent care.

What a sedation curriculum should look like

Not every institution is content with credentialing a non anesthesiologist provider with just the basic requirements, like ACLS. There are healthcare institutions that have nurses and physicians complete a certification program or curriculum before they can provide moderate sedation care. Frankly, that is how it should be. Not everybody is intuitive enough to provide safe moderate sedation without training.

Survey

There was a survey performed around 2000-2004 that is mentioned in Michael Kost's book, Moderate Sedation/Analgesia Core Competencies for Practice, that analyzes the hours of education non-anesthesia personnel administering conscious sedation received. Six hundred questionnaires went out to nurses and healthcare providers that administered moderate sedation to inpatients and outpatients. Of the six hundred, 275 responded. What they found was 60% of respondents replied in their questionnaire that they had received five hours or less of educational training and preparation for the administration and care of moderate sedation patients. The final conclusion to the survey demonstrated that few hours of moderate sedation training takes place and there is clearly a need for a standardized core curriculum [5]. It would be my best guess, based on the literature regarding the need for a standard core curriculum, that if another survey was sent out today the results would be similar.

Curriculums

One of the best curriculums I have seen comes from the Veteran Affairs (VA) National Center for Patient Safety. The VA National Center for Patient Safety has several publications, but the Moderate Sedation Toolkit for Non-Anesthesiologist, is by far one of the best curriculums available and should certainly be modeled after. What makes this curriculum first-class is its practically fool proof well organized format. This curriculum includes a facilitors guide, curriculum guide (box 3), pre-procedure templates, study guides, help cards, high fidelity simulation cases and table top cases [2].

Box 3 **VA Moderate Sedation Toolkit Curriculum Guide**

1. Pharmacology of commonly used medications
2. Relevant anatomy and physiology
3. Principles of pre-procedural patient assessment and education
4. Monitoring techniques
5. Required safety equipment
6. Common complications and their recognition and treatment
7. Special situations and high-risk patients

Another curriculum worth taking a peek at is the Multi-society Sedation Curriculum for Gastrointestinal Endoscopy (MSCGE). This Society has recognized the challenges of practicing gastroenterology face when dealing with moderate sedation by physician-nurse teams. Due to this assessment the MSCGE produced an 11 section curriculum (box 4) to serve as a guide for best practice. The curriculum was developed from expert opinions and evidence based practice [6].

Box 4
Multi-society Sedation Curriculum for Gastrointestinal Endoscopy (MSCGE)

1. Sedation Pharmacology
2. Informed consent
3. Peri-procedure assessment
4. levels of sedation
5. Training in the administration of special agents for moderate sedation

> 6. Training in airway/ rescue and management of complications
> 7. Anesthesiologist assistance for procedures
> 8. Intra-procedure monitoring
> 9. Post-procedure assessment training
> 10. Pregnant & lactating women
> 11. Assessment of competency

There are certainly a couple different curriculums circulating out there but it would be nice to see one standard curriculum, especially one that requires minimum training and education in the following areas:

1. Objective and goals of moderate sedation

2. Definitions of sedation levels

3. Informed consent for procedure and sedation

4. Regulatory bodies and organizations

5. Pre-procedure assessment

6. Pharmacology of commonly used medications

7. Intra-procedure monitoring and assessment

8. Required safety equipment

9. Common complications and their recognition and treatment

10. Special situations and high-risk patients

11. Post-procedure monitoring and assessment

12. Competency exam and simulation

There is a universal understanding that the specialty of moderate sedation is growing rapidly and it's hard to determine who is responsible for making standards and guidelines for the healthcare providers in this field. Perhaps one day a standardize curriculum for training and credentialing will be required by every healthcare institution as a gold standard for competency. In addition to a standard curriculum, there may also be a need for a stronger regulation on who can order and administer moderate sedation in the Untied States.

What can one do?

Even though there are healthcare organizations and states that require a healthcare provider to complete a curriculum for competency or privileges, there are just as many healthcare organizations in the United States that do not. So where do nurses turn if their institution and state offer little position nurses administering and managing adult moderate sedation? Well there are a few things that can be done to help a nurse under these circumstances:

- Get in contact with organizations that have recommendations on nursing and its role in sedation. There are organizations that spell out what a nurse is responsible for. For example the Association of Radiologic and Imaging Nursing, recommends that the intra-procedure nurse/monitor obtain and record vital signs every 5mins.

- Get involved in your institutions sedation team committee. If you don't know who to ask, go straight to the department of anesthesia. If there isn't a staff nurse that administers moderate sedation within the sedation committee, ask to be a member and represent your unit. Share your ideas on updating policies and practice. Even suggest a uniform training curriculum for physician-nurse teams within your institution. See if your institution will be willing to use this curriculum for credentialing.

- Ask your manager to get a few nurses within your department certified every year. Try these companies websites

    o **Sedation certification, Healthy Visions.** This group is magnet approved and recognized by **American Nurses Credentialing Center (ANCC).** They are also very helpful in answering any questions that you may have.

    o **Conscious sedation certification**
    http://www.conscioussedationcertification.com/index.html

- **Simsuite**
  http://www.medsimulation.com/ModerateSedation.asp

- **Conscious Sedation Consulting**
  http://www.sedationconsulting.com/ (this group will give sedation advice as well)

Become an active member in a few nationally recognized organizations like:

- *The American Association of Moderate Sedation Nurses (AAMSN)* http://aamsn.org/
- *Association of PeriOperative Registered Nurses (APORN)* http://www.aorn.org/
- *Association fro Radiologic and Imaging Nursing (ARIN)*
- *The Society of Gastroenterology Nurses and Associates, Inc. (SGNA)*
  - They offer Nursing Fellowship programs and Scholar programs for nurses based on evidence based practice. http://www.sgna.org/Home

The care of patients undergoing moderate sedation is relied upon state and federal compliance governing practice. Your state, CMS, and TJC all provide the basic credentialing requirements for those who can administrate and manage moderately sedated patients. It is then, the healthcare institutions responsibility to ensure that healthcare providers are competent to provide safe patient care. Unfortunately most healthcare institutions only strive for the basic requirements, such as ACLS or a rescue response team, to credential a healthcare provider. Perhaps one day we will see more stringent regulations on training and education in this specialized area.

Reference:

1. Department of Health & Human Services, Centers for Medicare & Medicaid Services. (2011). 482.52 conditions of participations: Anesthesia services (100-07). Retrieved from website:http://www.cms.gov/Regulations-and-Guidance/Guidance/Manuals/Internet-Only-Manuals-IOMs-Items/CMS1201984.html
2. The Durham VAMC Patient Safety Center of Inquiry (PSCI). (2011, march 29). Moderate sedation toolkit for non-anesthesiologists. Retrieved from http://www.patientsafety.gov/pubs.html
3. Eslinger, M. R. (n.d.). Moderate sedation certification. Retrieved from www.sedationcertification.com
4. The joint commission. (2012). Retrieved from http://www.jointcommission.org
5. Kost, M. (2004). Moderate sedation/analgesia. (2nd ed.). St. Louis: Saunders.
6. Splete, H. (2012, July 11). New sedation guideline sets in GI endoscopy. Internal Medicine News, Retrieved from http://internalmedicinenews.com
7. Urman, R. D, & Kaye, A. D. (2012). Moderate and deep sedation in clinical practice. New York Cambridge University Press.

Chapter 4

Pre-Procedure

Once you have reviewed your state laws, intuitional policies, and completed the necessary requirements to become qualified to administer moderate sedation, then you are able to understand what is required for safe and quality patient care in the pre-procedure, intra-procedure, and post procedure phases. Typically, each of these phases is broken down into three categories, Environment, Personnel, and Documentation. Due to the content this chapter will consist of only the pre-procedure phase.

The pre-procedural phase:

- is where the nurse and physician can gain vital information about the patient.
- Is when a sedation plan is developed.
- is the period when the patient is prepped for the procedure. Such as, antibiotics administration, intravenous line & Foley placement, and donning of hospital attire.
- Is the period when patient is assessed and documentation is verified.

See box 5 for TJC standards and requirements for pre-procedural phase

---

Box 5 — **TJC Standards**
PC.13.10, PC.13.20[4][9]

Environment

- Appropriate monitoring equipment is available.
- Appropriate equipment to administer fluids, drugs, blood and blood components is available.
- Resuscitation equipment is available

Personnel

- A registered nurse oversees peri-operative nursing care.
- A sufficient number of qualified staff is present, in addition to the healthcare provider performing the procedure, to assess the patient, provide the sedation, to assist with the procedure and to monitor and recover patient.
- The licensed physician with the privileges plans or concurs with the sedation plan.

> **Documentation**
> before moderate sedation procedure is performed:
> - a pre-sedation patient assessment is conducted
> - The patients anticipated needs are assessed in order to plan for post procedure care
> - Pre-procedural treatment and services are provided to the patients plan of care
> - Pre-procedural education, treatment and services are provided and discussed.
> - Pre-sedation evaluation and assessment completed.
> - A verification process such as a TIME OUT is utilized to confirm the site, procedure and patient prior to the start of the procedure.
> - 01.02.01 Marking of the procedure site.
>   - At a minimum, sites are marked when there is more than one possible location.
>   - Procedure site is marked by a licensed independent practitioner who is ultimately accountable for the procedure and will be present when the procedure is performed.
>   - A written, alternative process is in place for patients who refuse site marking or when it is technically or anatomically impossible to mark the site.
> - Immediately before moderate sedation is administered, the patient is re-evaluated. (This can occur in either the pre-procedure phase or the intra procedure phase).

Environment

Most institutions generally use pre anesthesia and same day care areas to prepare their patients for procedures requiring sedation. TJC, CMS and many other organizations do not stipulate where the pre-procedural phase occurs, but they do set guidelines and standards as to what has to occur in this period and by whom. Even if your institution doesn't utilize TJC, it wouldn't hurt to follow those guidelines. TJC has been reputable for helping hospitals become highly reliable organizations for developing "safe effective care" [10].

Personnel

The pre-procedure & intra-procedure nurse's duty is to ensure all documentation, labs and tests are collected and completed prior to the procedure. The pre-procedure nurse acts as the first line gate keeper. Neither sedation nor procedure should start until the nurse affirms that the appropriate pre-procedure documentation is completed. Any incomplete documentation and abnormal tests must be addressed by this nurse. All team members involved in the pre-evaluation are held accountable for identifying incomplete documentation and high risk patients (based on their assessment and pre-evaluation documentation). If a patient's physical status is considered high risk for complications (ASA 3 or above), then anesthesia should be consulted [12].

Box 9 Identifies responsibilities of the physician and the nurse. It is not outside a nurse's scope of practice to perform an ASA assessment or a Mallampati airway exam.

Box 9	Responsibilies	
Documentation	Licensed Independent Practitioner(LIP) Responsibility	Nurse Responsibility (According to AORN & ARIN)
Patient Interview	Legal	Strongly Recommended
Physical Exam	Legal	Strongly Recommended
ASA physical classification & Mallampati Airway exam	Strongly Recommended	Strongly Recommended
Chart Review	Legal	Strongly Recommended
Reference: Association of Peri-Operative Registered Nurses (AORN) & Association for Radiologic & Imaging Nursing (ARIN)		

What happens if the nurse's assessment differs from the LIP's?

If by chance the nurse's evaluation differs from the privileged physician, than here are a few suggestions (also see decision tree in appendix):

- The nurse should collaborate with the physician they are teamed with and verbalize their patient's assessment differed from his or hers. If the nurse feels as though the patient is at high risk for complications, then that nurse should be sure to back up his/or her assessment with legitimate evidence.

- Some physicians may respect the nurse's assessment and agree while others may not be so agreeable. If a physician doesn't agree with the nurse's evaluation then trying approaches of persuasion and compromise:

    I. Politely offer the physician with an alternative plan, such as obtaining an anesthesia consult, anti antiemetic therapy, naso-gastric tube placement, CPAP machine etc. It is important that the nurse show the LIP that he or she wants the patient to have their procedure done, but in a safe manner [8].

    II. Reproach: If the LIP does not agree, give some time and reproach with other solutions or reasoning. People are more receptive to grant your request after they declined the first one. They will feel embarrassed, especially if it's much easier to comply than the first request [8].

- Nurses are the "last line of defense, the patient advocate, the defender and the gate keeper" [4]. The nurse may need to be assertive. It is however important to not become angry or defensive. Most of all a nurse should not feel guilty for protecting the patient and his/her licensure.

- The nurse should use polite friendly words such as

    I. "Mr. K has COPD, CHF, and ejection fraction of 15% and wears a Bipap at night. I do not feel comfortable sedating this patient. I believe he is beyond my scope of practice and would receive better care under anesthesia services at this time."

II. "The patient is showing EKG changes and I no longer feel comfortable continuing the procedure without further evaluation..."

- The nurse should demonstrate confidence but refrain from being arrogant [8].

If the nurse is still having trouble convincing the physician they are teamed with that providing moderate sedation is not the safest practice for the patient based upon their assessment, than other steps may include:

- Getting management involved.
- Exercising nursing rights via The Nurse Practice Act.
  - As a moderate sedation nurse administrating medications, it is the nurse's obligation to protect the patient. If there is a realistic, reasonable and individualized evaluation by the nurse that injury or death could occur from administrating this particular medication, than the nurse has the right to withhold the medication [3].
- Refuse the patient assignment
  - If the patient assignment is beyond the nurse's skill level and then this would be an example of an inappropriate delegation by the physician [4]. Every nurse providing moderate sedation should be able to recognize those patients who are at risk for complications. This nurse has the right to say he/she is not adequately trained to sedate this particular patient. With this said there should be no pressure forced upon this nurse to sedate a patient who does not fit the appropriate criteria for moderate sedation.

Documentation

The purpose of the pre-procedural assessment is to identify and mange risks associated with moderate sedation and the procedure it's self. CMS requires the procedural physician to participate in the pre-procedure evaluation [12].This process should start from when the physician first meets the patient up until the immediate start of the procedure [11].

Most non legal organizations such as the American Association of Nurse Anesthetists (AANA), ASA, AORN, ARIN, and SGNA, share similar recommendations on what should be documented and evaluated before a patient receives sedation. Below are recommended guidelines for pre-procedure evaluation and documentation from AORN, ASA, TJC and CMS requirements for the pre-procedure phase.

PATIENT INTERVIEW

1. Age, Height, Weight
2. Vital signs
3. Allergies
4. ETHOL/Substance abuse
5. Level of Consciousness
6. NPO status (as per ASA guidelines)

- Aspiration may occur intra-procedure from moderate sedation in patients who enter a state of deep sedation and have lost their protective airway reflexes [9].
  - NPO guidelines rarely mention oral contrast. As, per a study conducted in 2010, on Gastric emptying time of oral contrast material in children and adolescents undergoing abdominal computed tomography, concluded that a patient should be NPO for 3hrs after ingesting oral contrast [2].
  - The ASA Sedation Model Policy stated that certain radiological procedures require the administration of oral fluids in conjunction with sedation and analgesia. Risk of aspiration during these

procedures must be weighed against the benefits of sedation and analgesia. Patients undergoing these types of procedures must be informed of risks. The following is not a recommendation but a suggestion: In the event that the NPO requirements are adjusted, the credentialed physician may administer moderate sedation with operating monitoring personnel and appropriate documentation to include rationale must be included in the medical record [9].

7. Responsible adult escort

    o   This is someone over the age of 18, who can receive and understand instructions, stay with the patient for 24 hours, and call for assistance [1] [9].

8. Menstrual history/pregnancy

9. Pain

    o   While there isn't a specific Joint Commission standard that prescriptively mandates the assessment of pain during moderate sedation cases, this is a practice adopted by many organizations to ensure adequate sedation and analgesia is achieved during procedures. This information then may be used as a metric in evaluating any adverse events related to sedation or anesthesia (see PI.01.01.01 EP 6) as well as evaluating the practitioner's ability to effectively manage moderate sedation patients (see MS.08.01.03 and PC.03.01.01 EP 1). It is important to keep in mind that the requirements found at PC.01.02.07 regarding pain assessment and management should not be 'excluded' from procedures or procedural areas as patients have a right to have their pain managed while receiving any care, treatment or service.

    o   SGNA recommends-baseline pain assessment using institutionally approved pain scale with identification of area, duration and type of pain [6].

- The American Society for Pain Management Nursing (ASPMN) recommends that before, during and after procedures, pain should be assessed and managed [5].
  - Patients with acute or chronic pain may be controlling their pain with anxiolytics, antidepressants, anticonvulsants, muscle relaxants, pumps (PCA & internal) and nerve stimulators. Unless an adverse reaction is foreseen these treatments should not be discontinued [12].

10. A Physical exam

- Heart
  - Assessment of rhythm, ejection fraction, murmurs etc.
  - The American College of Cardiology (ACC) and the American Heart Association (AHA) task force report guidelines for peri-operative Cardiovascular Evaluation for NON cardiac surgeries. The ACC and the AHA suggest that non-cardiac surgery before 6 weeks after a myocardial infarction is considered high risk, and an intermediate risk for non-cardiac surgery before 3 months [11]. If an infarction does reoccur, the mortality rate is roughly 50% [9]
- Lung/airway
  - Sounds
  - Mallampati Airway Classification System (box 6)
    - Primarily performed by physician, however nurses can perform as well.
    - COPD, Emphysema, asthma, sleep Apnea
      - This population is sensitive to respiratory depressant effects [9].
      - Morphine is contraindicated in asthmatic patients due to its histamine releasing properties [9].

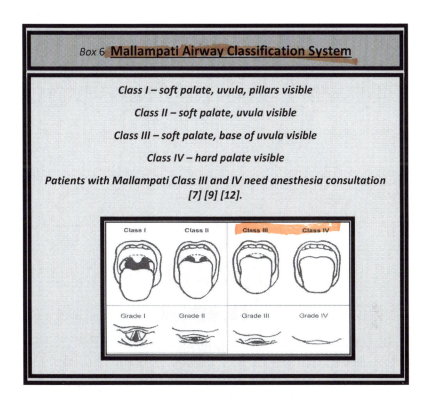

Box 6 **Mallampati Airway Classification System**

Class I – soft palate, uvula, pillars visible

Class II – soft palate, uvula visible

Class III – soft palate, base of uvula visible

Class IV – hard palate visible

Patients with Mallampati Class III and IV need anesthesia consultation [7] [9] [12].

- Endocrine [9]
    - Those patients with diabetes and taking oral hypoglycemic need to hold their medication and should have their procedure scheduled in the morning.
    - Glucose levels should be checked immediately prior to procedure and also during post procedure.
    - Some physicians prefer metformin to be held for 2 days post procedure especially when dye is used intravenously or intra-arterially.
- Neuro status
- Hepatic
    - Those patients with acute or chronic liver failure are at risk for arterial de-saturation, electrolyte disturbances, and poor metabolism of pharmacologic compounds dependent of hepatic blood flow and enzyme activity [9].
        - Gastrointestinal
        - Renal

- o Those patients with acute or chronic renal failure are at risk for acidosis, fluid overload, hypertension, renal clearance and electrolyte imbalances [9].
- o Record of last date of dialysis should be noted in chart [9].
- Musculosketel
- Integumentary
- Anesthesia/ surgical History
- Lab Data
    - o Are not required but should be used to foresee any complications, decrease morbidity and mortality.
- A completed physical status classification from the American Society of Anesthesiologists (ASA) based on assessment see box 7.

Box 7

ASA 1
A normally healthy patient. e.g.
No chronic illness, no regular medications

ASA 2
A patient with mild systemic disease.
e.g. Controlled hypertension and Type II Diabetes. History of tobacco use. Obesity, Non-metastatic carcinoma. A well-controlled asthma patient with no recent exacerbations. A child with underlying cerebral palsy. A child with a well-controlled seizure disorder.

ASA 3
A patient with severe systemic disease. e.g.
Poorly controlled hypertension. Multiple medications for cardiac, respiratory and/or metabolic disorders. Metastatic disease with some interference with function. Pneumonia
This may be divided into STABLE and UNSTABLE categories:
Stable: Controlled insulin-dependent diabetic with hypertension and mild renal disease. A child with congenital heart disease stable on digoxin and lasix.
Unstable: Frequent asthma attacks needing ER visits or intubation. Brittle, or difficult to control, insulin dependent diabetic. Severe COPD, on multiple inhalers and difficulty breathing in supine position

> **ASA 4**
> A patient with severe systemic disease that is a constant threat to life. e.g.
> Metastatic disease with severe organ dysfunction. Severe hypertension with angina.
> <u>Recent MI</u> with continuing symptoms.
> Sepsis, organ insufficiency
>
> **ASA 5**
> A moribund patient who is not expected to survive. e.g.
> Poorly responsive cardiogenic shock.
>
> Ruptured Abdominal Aortic Aneurysm with severe hypotension. Head trauma with increasing ICP

CHART REVIEW

1. Past medical history
2. Surgical history
3. lab studies (include pregnancy 8-55 yrs of age)
4. Current medications
    - including anticoagulants, sleeping medications, tranquilizers and over-the-counter drugs, herbal agents or illicit drugs [9].
5. Ancillary studies (EKG)
6. NPO status
    - As per ASA guidelines
7. Code Status (as per ASPAN) [1]
    - This is often never discussed. Occasionally, patients with NO CPR orders undergo procedures with different levels of sedation, ranging from moderate to general. Because the administration of sedation can cause cardiac and respiratory depression that may lead to cardiac and respiratory arrest that is typically reversible, patients who have NO CPR orders may not want CPR withheld, esp. if it is brought on by sedation. It is therefore necessary for a physician treating a pt with a DNR or NO CPR to re-discuss the

patient's resuscitation status. If agreed upon by pt, temp suspension of NO CPR should occur until after pt has recovered from sedation. Discussion of status should be documented in Patient's medical chart or included on the inform consent [1].

8. Consent obtained (procedure & sedation)
   - It is generally the credentialed healthcare provider performing the procedure, responsibility to obtain the pre-procedure documentation. However, midlevel practitioners, fellows and residents can as well [12]. Nurses are not to obtain consents; they can however verify the patient's understanding and the completion of the consents.
   - A lack of appropriately obtained informed consents may constitute charges of assault and battery [8].
   - Informed consent must address risks, benefits and alternatives. However every institutions consent form are different. Many institutions will include the pre-procedure evaluation along with the risks, benefits and alternatives.
     - See form in box 8 for an example of a consent form

Box 8   Moderate Sedation Consent Form Example
front

Date____/____/____

Pre-Procedure Evaluation
Age:___ Sex:___ wt:___ Ht:___ B/P:___ P:___ R:___ O2sat:___ Temp:___
Allergies:_____
Current Medications:_____
Previous reaction to sedation: Yes____ No ____ describe:_____
Family History of reaction to anesthesia: Yes ____ No:_____
describe:_____
   ASA Classification:_____ Mallampati Airway Classification:_____
        H&P on chart and reviewed within last 24 hrs:
                Yes :____ No:___
   History & Physical   Inpatient: _____ H&P on chart _____

Outpatient:

H&P Completed within 30 days Yes____NO____ Complete below
Past Medical History:_____
Surgical HX:_____
Lungs:_____Heart:_____Skin:____ General Appearance:_____
Additional Findings:_____
Pregnant: Yes NO   Tobacco: Yes NO describe:_____ETOH: Yes NO
describe:_____
Recreational Drugs: Yes   NO
describe:_____
EKG: Yes NO N/A   CXR : YES NO N/A   NPO: Yes NO
Last oral intake:_____
Acute Chronic Scale: _____   Score:____ Comfort Level:_____
Describe:_____

Back of Form

Sedation Plan

Moderate _____ Deep_____Anesthesia consult _____
Patient is an appropriate candidate for the planned procedure and sedation: Yes NO
Physician Signature:_____Date: ___/___/____Time:_____
Consent   N/A if patient has airway protection and already on sedation

I, _____, acknowledge that the physician performing the procedure has explained to me that I will have sedation/analgesia services provided during my procedure. I am aware that the type of sedation/analgesia that is used is based upon the type of procedure, my medical and physical condition, doctor's preference and my own decision. I have been informed that there are risks from being sedated, and there are no guarantees that complications may not arise. I have been informed that the sedation provided may cause me to experience cardiac, respiratory and paradoxical reactions that may require me to receive reversal medications, advance cardiac and respiratory support. Risks, alternatives and expected benefits have been explained to me in layman's terms. All my questions have been answered at this time.

Patient or guardian's signature :_____Date:__/__/__ Time:___
Physician signature:_____ Date:__/__/___ Time:___
Witness:_____Date:___/__/____Time:_____
The Patient is unable to consent because_____

The principle of the pre-procedure evaluation is to establish a rapport with the patient but more importantly discover whether the patient fits into the criteria for moderate sedation. This can be done through a thorough review of the patient's history and physical assessment. If the pre-procedure evaluation is not completed or performed correctly the patient may endure complications from the procedure or sedation. Not only does this constitute unsafe practice, but if litigation occurs, the malpractice attorney with the lawsuit will address the inadequacy of pre-procedure assessment. So in conclusion, Knowing your role as either the pre or intra-procedure nurse is very imperative in the moderate sedation plan process. They are considered the role of the frontline gatekeeper and should not settle for mediocre care. The nurses owe the patient the duty of taking the time to evaluate that the pre-procedure assessment and evaluation are done right!

Reference:

1. American Society of PeriAnesthesia Nurses. (2012-2014). *Perianesthesia nursing standards, practice recommendations and interpretive statements*. American Society of PeriAnesthesia Nurses.
2. Berger-Achituv, S., Zissin, R., Shenkman, Z., Gutermaker, M., & Erez, I. (2010). Gastric emptying time of oral contrast material in children and adolescents undergoing abdominal computed tomography. JPGN, 51, 31-34. Retrieved from www.jpgn.org
3. Brent, N. J. (n.d.). When does a nurse have the right to refuse to give a patient medication? [Online forum comment]. Retrieved from Nurse.com
4. Brooke, P. S. (2009, July). Legally speaking. when can you say no?. Nursing 2013, 39(7), 42-46. Retrieved fromhttp://www.nursingcenter.com
5. Czarnecki, M., Turner, H., Collins, P., Doellman, D., Wrona, S., & Reynolds, J. (2011). Procedural pain management: A position statement with clinical practice . doi: 1524-9042
6. Education Committee of the Society of Gastroenterology Nurses and Associates, Inc. (SGNA) chaired by Trina Van Guilder, RN,BSN,CGRN. (2003). Guidelines for documentation in. Retrieved from http://www.sgna.org/Portals/0/Education/Practice Guidelines/DocumentationGuideline.pdf

7. ESLINGER, M. R. (n.d.). Moderate sedation certification. Retrieved from www.sedationcertification.com
8. Lee, A. 21 powerful ways to persuade people to do. Retrieved from http://www.20daypersuasion.com/21WaysToPersuade.pdf
9. Kost, M. (2004). Moderate sedation/analgesia. (2nd ed.). St. Louis: Saunders.
10. Meldi, D., Rhoades, F. & Gippe, A. (2009, 01). The big three: A side by side matrix comparing hospital accrediting agencies. Synergy, 14-16. Retrieved from http://www.hfap.org/mediacenter/NAMSS Synergy JanFeb09_Accreditation Grid.pdf
11. (2009). Patient screening and assessment in ambulatory surgical facilities. Pennsylvania Patient Safety advisory, 6(1), 3-8.
12. The joint commission. (2012). Retrieved from http://www.jointcommission.org
13. Urman, R. D, & Kaye, A. D. (2012). Moderate and deep sedation in clinical practice. New York: Cambridge University Press.

Chapter 5

Intra-Procedure

The intra-procedure phase is the most climatic and critical period of adult moderate sedation. While the goals and objectives of moderate sedation are significant, safety is the number one priority. During this phase, the patient is completely vulnerable to the person administrating the sedation and the physician providing the procedure. Whether sedation occurs in the Emergency Department, Operating Room, MRI, CT scan, Endoscopy, Radiology or Cath Lab Suites, the required personnel, documentation, and environment all need to be consistent and compliant with regulatory bodies, throughout the healthcare institution (see TJC standards in box 10).

Box 10 — ***TJC***
Standard PC 13.20, 13.30 & Chapter National Safety Goals 01.01.01, 01.02.01, 01.03.01, 03.04.0, PI 01.01.01 [12][13]

Environment

- Appropriate equipment to monitor the patient's physiologic status is available.
- Appropriate equipment to administer intravenous fluids and drugs, including blood and blood components, is available as needed.
- Resuscitation capabilities are available.
- Appropriate methods are used to continuously monitor oxygenation, ventilation, and circulation during procedures that may affect the patient's physiological status.

Personnel

- A sufficient number of qualified staff is present, in addition to the healthcare provider performing the procedure, to assess the patient, provide the sedation, to assist with the procedure and to monitor and recover patient.
- Individuals administering moderate sedation are qualified and have appropriate credentials to manage patients at whatever level of sedation or anesthesia is achieved, either intentionally or unintentionally.

Documentation

- The patient is re-evaluated immediately before moderate sedation and before anesthesia induction.
- The procedure and/or administration of sedation for each patient are documented in the medical chart.

- 01.03.01 TIME OUT –a designated member of the team initiates the time out and it includes active communication among all relevant members of the procedure team.

    TIME OUT INCLUDES:
    o **CORRECT PATIENT IDENTITY**
    o **CORRECT SITE**
    o **CORRECT PROCEDURE**

- When one or more procedures are being performed on the same patient, and the person performing the procedure changes, perform a TIME OUT before each procedure is initiated.
- 01.02.01 **Marking of the procedure site.**
    o At a minimum, sites are marked when there is more than one possible location.
    o Procedure site is marked by a licensed independent practitioner who is ultimately accountable for the procedure and will be present when the procedure is performed.
    o A written, alternative process is in place for patients who refuse site marking or when it is technically or anatomically impossible to mark the site.
- PI 01.01.01 **The hospital collects data to monitor its performance**. The hospital collects data on the following:
    - The results of resuscitation
    - Significant adverse drug reactions

Environment

The environment a nurse sedates in plays a very important part in safety. The room should be large enough for the physician, and for the nurse to assist the physician and patient. The nurse must be able to maneuver around the room especially to assess ventilatory and airway access. In addition TJC speciation's, the room needs to be in compliance with other regulating bodies like OSHA.

Not only does the room have to be large enough to work in but appropriate equipment must be in place and in working order before any moderate sedation case begins. The following is the list of required equipment that needs to be readily available and in working order:

o Oxygen
o Ambu bag with appropriate mask
o Oxygen therapy devices
o Nasal cannula, non-rebreather, etc.

- Extension tubing and connectors
- Oral & Nasal adjuncts
- Obturator available for tracheostomy patient
- continuing monitoring devices for ventilatory, cardiac and oxygen status.
- Suction
- With appropriate suction catheters available
- Reversal drugs
- Preferably in your possession

Personnel

The personnel generally involved in moderate sedation cases include, but are not limited to:

1. ***The credentialed/privileged physician*** conducting the procedure and ordering the moderate sedation medication.

    a. **ASA task force practice guidelines for non-anesthesiologists states [13]:**

        i. Healthcare providers responsible for patients receiving moderate sedation should understand the pharmacology of moderate sedation agents and their antagonists.

2. ***A non-anesthetist,*** qualified personnel in airway rescue and sedation administration, who administers the medication and monitors the patient's physiologic status under the supervision of a credentialed/privileged physician [21].

a. *Depending on your state this can be:*
    i. Radiology technologist
    ii. A midlevel practitioner, such as a Radiology assistant
    iii. Nurse

    - **ASA task force practice guidelines for non-anesthesiologists states [13]:**

        - A designated health care provider other than the physician performing the procedure should be present to monitor the patient throughout the procedure performed with moderate sedation.

- The health care provider monitoring patients receiving moderate sedation should be able to recognize complications. At least one individual should be able to summon for help and establish a patent airway and deliver positive pressure ventilation. It is recommended that healthcare personnel with ACLS skills be in the immediate area when moderate sedation is being delivered.

3. **An assistant to the physician** for the case [13].

    a. *Radiology technologist, nurse, medical assistant, surgical assistant, physician assistant, etc*

Every institution may differ in the personnel that are utilized within a procedure room for a moderate sedation case. Here are some examples of moderate sedation teams:

- A staff physician (a resident and/or fellow if credentialed and overseen by staff physician) to perform the procedure and order moderate sedation.

- A nurse, technologist, resident and or physician assistant- to assist with equipment and scrub.

- a radiology technologist maneuvers and operates the radiology machinery.

- and a nurse, radiology technologist or midlevel provide moderate sedation and monitor the patient.

The Nurse

Regardless of the personnel that are used within a moderate sedation case, they need to meet state and federal regulations, and institutional policies. The appropriate personnel should also have or be provided with the right training and education in order to administer moderate sedation safety to a patient. Generally speaking, a registered nurse is probably the most widely used personnel privileged to administer moderate sedation under the direct supervision of a credentialed physician. Perhaps this is because of their training and approach to patient care differs from other health care providers. Nurses receive extensive training and education in ethics, advocacy, spirituality, disease processes, pharmacology, and the promotion and optimization of health and wellness. There is simply a more extensive role for nurses than just data collection in moderate sedation.

> Nursing as per the American Nurses Association (ANA), is the protection, promotion, and optimization of health and abilities, prevention of illness and injury, alleviation of suffering through the diagnosis and treatment of human response, and advocacy in the care of individuals, families, communities, and populations [2].

Training

Besides the fact that a nurse needs a degree in nursing, state licensure, and credentialing through their institutions, there are several additional qualifications and training that nationally recognized organizations, who have position statements on moderate sedation by a nurse, wish for a nurse to possess. For instance **The American Association of Moderate Sedation Nurses**, founded in 2008, states the following position about nurses providing moderate sedation.

"Registered nurses must have the knowledge and experience with medications used and skills to assess, interpret and intervene in the event of complications. This registered nurse is an asset to the physician and enhances the quality of care provided to the patient" .

The American Society of Peri-Anesthesia Nursing is another organization that states the following [3]:

The administration of IV moderate sedation medications by non-anesthetist RN's are allowed by state law and institutional policy/protocol.

The RN managing the care of the patient during the procedure, while giving IV moderate sedation, should have no other responsibilities that would leave the patient unattended or compromise continuous monitoring.

The nurse administering moderate sedation must also be able to [10][11][13][14][19]:

- Understand and demonstrate the ability to use oxygen delivery devices.
- Anticipate and identify possible complications of IV moderate sedation in relation to the type of medication being dispensed.
- Assess respiratory rate, oxygen saturation, blood pressure, cardiac rate, and rhythm and patient's level of consciousness.
- Possess the knowledge and skills to assess, diagnose, and intervene in the event of complications. The nurse must also able to provide nursing interventions in compliance with orders or institutional protocols and guidelines.
  - Demonstrate skill in airway management resuscitation.
  - ***Should have no other responsibilities*** other than administering medications and monitoring the patient's physiologic status . However, the ASA recommends if the nurse is asked to help in a minor task the patient must be stable. Keep in mind that accepting any additional task may compromise patient safety and the nurse has the right to refuse any additional tasks during this period if he or she feels the patient is unstable[4] .
  - Demonstrates knowledge of the legal consequence or administering moderate sedation and/or monitoring patients receiving moderate sedation, including the responsibilities and liabilities of the RN in the event of an life-threatening complication [14].

Role

The role of nurse administering moderate sedation spans beyond just hands on training, which is why they tend to stand out amongst other healthcare providers. Some of the most important roles a moderate sedation may function as include the caregiver, educator, protector, and advocator.

The Caregiver Role

The caregiver role is the most traditional role that provides direct care and promotes comfort [16]. This role fosters nurturing and compassion characteristics which are very appreciated even in a moderate sedation setting. Some important examples of how this role can help in moderate sedation cases included but are not limited to:

- Include the patient in conversations

"Words are, of course, the most powerful drug used by mankind."- Rudyard Kipling [11].

   - The influence of words and distraction are sometimes the most powerful tools:

      - When a person is isolated, they have plenty of time alone to invoke troublesome thoughts that can make them anxious, by socializing with your patient, their anxieties take a back seat and they begin to relax [9][11]. By reducing fear and anxiety of the patient, there is less stress on the cardiovascular system, and vasovagal reactions are less likely to occur [9][18].

      - Florence Nightingale directed nurses to use words to help patients to change their thoughts. Words are still the most powerful tool a nurse has. For instance Negative thoughts/words can induce individuals to have a sickening feeling and positive thoughts/words can make individuals feel well. So, when your patient is in the room avoid words like, 'needles,' 'pain,' 'blood,' and instead use words like 'uncomfortable,' 'comfortable,' 'pressure,' and the phrase "I'll be with you the whole time" [11].

The Educator Role

The educator role provides the patient with information about the procedure and moderate sedation. Educating the patient on the expectations and process involved in prepping and preparing for the procedure while intra-procedure can alleviate anxiety. It is also important that introduction of those individuals in the procedure room are known and explanations of the expectations of the moderate sedation are conveyed. This role can re-enforce a good rapport.

The Protector Role

The protector Role is more or less defensive type of nursing. Nurses simply ensure patient safety and intervene In the event of complications. They do so by promoting morally and ethically sound decisions and tasks.

The Advocator Role

The advocator role involves the concern and actions in behalf of the patient to bring about a change [18]. In this role the moderate sedation nurse can promote what is best for the patient, ensuring that the patient's needs are met and their rights are protected. The nurse also provides explanations in language that patients understand and supports the decisions the patient makes.

Because of these unique roles, nurses differ from other healthcare providers. They simply must have a great amount of autonomy, assertiveness, ability to troubleshoot, and think far in advance in order to provide and care for a moderately sedated patient. The moderate sedation nurse must have experience in pharmacology of medications that are given, and must know the affects of those medications on their patient's poly-pharmacy and complex co-morbities. Most times because of these advance skills nurses with critical care experience, tend to make the best moderate sedation nurses [11][16][17].

Documentation

TJC does not specifically required a standard set of documentation for moderate sedation but rather leave this responsibility to each healthcare organization to determine their own documentation format [12].

The following box 11 is an example list of documentation that should be completed during the intra procedure phase:

| Box 11 | **Documentation during the Intra- Procedure Phase** |

Checklist of tasks
- Consents obtained
- Emergency supplies available and functional
- Oxygen
- Suction
- History, physical, labs, medications reviewed

TIME OUT!

Patent IV Access

Physiologic monitoring equipment used and assessment
- Pulse Oximeter
- Capnography (not required)
- EKG
- Temperature (only if indicated)
- Blood pressure
- Oxygen
- Level of Conscious/sedation
- Pain

Medications

Surgical Wounds and line placements

Pre-Post Aldrete score

Start and stop of procedure

Outcome measures tool
- Process & Patient Outcome

Checklist of tasks

Because the intra-procedure nurse is responsible for ensuring safety and sedation level, he or she must make certain that all the pre-procedure verification is completed. Generally this is done by receiving report from the pre-procedure nurse and assessment of the patient. However, not all institutions use pre-op areas to verify patient readiness, especially for inpatients. In instances like these it is then the responsibility of the intra-procedure nurse to verify all consents, labs, and any other important information pertaining to the patient and procedure.

So, before the procedure starts the intra procedure nurse is responsible for:

- Receiving a nurse report from pre-procedure nurse or bedside nurse.
    - Did the patient receive any ordered antibiotics?
    - Did the patient receive premedication for Iodine contrast allergy?
    - Were abnormal labs addressed? And so on...
- Ensuring that the pre-procedure checklist is verified and completed.
    - Labs
    - EKG
    - NPO Status etc....
- Ensuring that consents are completed.
    - If not the procedure needs to be delayed until this legal documentation is completed.
- Ensuring that patient is a good candidate for moderate sedation.
    - Completing a quick but thorough assessment of patient.
    - Keep in mind, the nurse administrating the moderate sedation can refuse to except the assignment if he or she feels that:
        - there is a realistic, reasonable and individualized evaluation by the nurse that injury or death could occur from administrating this particular medication [3].
        - The patient assignment is beyond the nurse's skill level and this can be an inappropriate delegation by the physician [4]. Every nurse providing moderate sedation should be able to recognize those patients who are at risk for complications. This nurse has the right to say he/she is not adequately trained to sedate this particular

patient. With this said there should be no pressure forced upon this nurse to sedate a patient who does not fit the appropriate criteria for moderate sedation.

- **TIME OUT**

> **TIME OUT INCLUDES:**
> **CORRECT PATIENT IDENTITY**
> **CORRECT SITE**
> **CORRECT PROCEDURE**

  - Don't assume other individuals in the room have already done this. Always verify patient identification.
  - The nurse can perform this task but the TIME OUT can be initiated by anyone and is best done when everybody involved in the procedure, is in the room and ready to start the procedure [12].
  - When one or more procedures are being performed on the same patient, and the person performing the procedure changes, perform a TIME OUT before each procedure is initiated.

- **Pre and Post Anesthesia Scoring System** [14]
  - Performed by the nurse in the pre and post procedure phases. Some institutions may require that this be performed before the patient leaves a moderate sedation procedure room especially if a patient does not recover in a post sedation recovery area.
  - Some healthcare institutions may use this system as a means to assessing the patient's level of functioning but this system was developed for assessing the patient's readiness to discharge and is not recommended as a scale to measure a patient's level of sedation [14][19].
  - The Aldrete was introduced in clinical practice in 1970. It is probably the most widely used scoring system until development of the Modified Aldrete (see box 12) [19].

Box 12 Aldrete[14][19]	Modified Aldrete [14][19]
Activity	Activity
Respiration	Respiration
Circulation	Circulation
Consciousness	Consciousness
Oxygen Saturation	Oxygen Saturation
	Dressing
	Pain
	Ambulation
	Fasting-Feeding
	Urine Output
Based on score of 10	Based on score of 20

- **Surgical Wounds, Line Placements and Removals**
    - Documentation of any lines and surgical wounds added during the procedure should be placed in the patient's chart. This may included but is not limited to:
        - Sheaths, Arterial lines, central lines, biopsy site, catheter insertion site.
    - Documentation and assessment of any line and tube removals should also be included in the patient's chart.

- **Medications**
    - Moderate sedation medications should be ordered prior to the start of the procedure by the credentialed physician performing the procedure.
    - Documentation of medications given, time, route and frequency, should be included in the patient's chart.
- **Patent IV Access**
    - Preferably 20 gauge or larger and patent
- **Physiologic monitoring** devices and assessment

- Monitoring should be tailored to specific procedure, patient factors, medical conditions and type of sedation to be administered [19].

> The American Radiologic and Imaging Nursing (ARIN) recommends that vital signs be taken and documented every 5 min. and at one minute after each additional dose of IV sedative.

1. **Pulse Oximeter**
    - Repetitive research shows that pulse ox probes placed on the patient's ear are more accurate and have quicker response times, than probes placed anywhere else on the body [13][14].
    - In cases when oxygen saturation is below 65%, the monitoring device generally over calculates and provide a false reading [13][14].

2. **Capnography** (net yet required for moderate sedated patients, but is becoming a national standard for many organizations)(see Capnography in Appendix)
    - Provides information on ventilation. Sometimes EKG leads are not placed in the ideal position for monitoring ventilation effectively. Capnography allows early detection of hypoventilation and possible airway obstructions [7][13][14].
    - Normal Capnography Values ETCO2 35-45mmHg. Imperfect positioning of nasal cannula capno-filters, mouth breathers and nasal obstructions can distort reading. Also O2 via mask can lower readings by 10% [7].
    - Not commonly used in moderate sedation cases but may prove beneficial in patients:
        - have their heads covered by sterile drapes.
        - that are positioned prone.
        - that are ICU patients, intubated and are already on sedation drips.

3. **EKG** [13][14]
   - Depending on the procedure, your placement of EKG leads may differ from the norm. The idea is however, to get the best wave form as possible. The best leads to monitor in are Lead II and V5 or MCL in a 3 lead EKG.
   - Lead II provides a waveform easily identified and preferred by most health care providers. Allows easy visualization of P waves and arrhythmias, but difficult to see bundle branch blocks [13][14].
   - Lead V5 or MCL in 3 lead, is the preferred lead for detecting myocardial ischemia (MI) [13][14][17].
     - T-wave inversion is seen first in patients having an MI. The T- wave becomes tall and peaked with a wide base.
     - ST segment becomes elevated = myocardial injury.
     - Most common arrhythmias are premature ventricular complexes (PVC) and atrial dysrhythmias.
     - Most arrhythmias/dysrhythmais occur secondary to hypoxia, which is reversed by oxygen therapy.
   - The interpretation of leads and waveforms is imperative for the moderate sedation nurse. Every nurse providing sedation should be able to recognize changes in the patient's condition and if extenuating circumstances arise the nurse is confident and comfortable intervening. It is the nurse's duty to be able to identify these changes and report to the physician he or she is working under.
4. **Temperature** (only if indicated)
5. **Blood pressure**
   - Invasive or non-invasive

6. **Oxygen**
    - This is controversial. Some physicians prefer their patients be on oxygen prior to sedation while other physicians use this as an intervention only [14]. I would have to say this would be a question for the sedation committee in your institution. There should be a monitoring tool to measure patient outcomes from moderate sedation under a credentialed physician. In this tool it may ask you if you had to apply oxygen to the patient for an O2 Sat less than 10% of the patient's baseline. If so than I would say this was an intervention.

7. **Level of Conscious**
    - To make certain that the goals of moderate sedation are being met, the nurse should assess the level of sedation by using a sedation scale. There are many different scales available [13][14]. The Ramsay Scale, Observer's Assessment of alertness/Sedation, Sedation Visual Analogue Scale are some examples. The BIS monitor may also be helpful, but is likely not seen in moderate sedation cases[13][14].
        - Monitored at least every 15 min [13][14].
        - Restless and agitation should always be considered signs of hypoxemia until proven otherwise [14].

8. **Pain** [1][4][8][15][16][17][20]
    - This seems to be a controversial subject. Should a patient's pain level be assessed during moderate sedation? There is little literature on this topic supporting either side. The argument here is, as a moderate sedation nurse, are you going to walk to the head of bed and wake the patient from their moderately sedated state to assess their pain level? Especially during procedures that require little movement as possible. You wouldn't have a patient wake up

and talk in the middle of brain surgery, so how do moderate sedated procedures differ?

It certainly seems like a pain assessment during the procedure would defeat the purpose of moderately sedation if we conducted pain assessments during a procedure. But we have to keep in mind that the goal of moderate sedation is not sleeping, but providing relief of anxiety and pain for the patient. With this said it would be an unreasonable failure on our part as healthcare providers to not recognized and treat pain during a moderately sedated procedure. This would certainly be viewed by a moral and legal stand point as an unethical breach of human rights. So let's look at some of the position statements given by nationally recognized organizations:

- TJC requires that all patients be assessed for pain and have their pain controlled appropriately [12].
- SGNA recommends-baseline pain assessment using institutionally approved pain scale with identification of area, duration and type of pain [10].
- The American Society for Pain Management Nursing (ASPMN) recommends that before, during and after procedures, pain should be assessed and managed. Pain and anxiety should be assessed if the patient is awake during the procedure [4][8].
- The World Health Organization (WHO) views pain relief as a basic human right [4][8].

Even though the argument is very strong supporting the importance of assessing and managing pain during a moderate sedation procedure, there seems to be little guidelines offered on how to implement this practice . This basically leaves your institution to gather information and formulate a process, policy and procedure for this subject.

Helpful Suggestions:

o Pain should be assessed immediately prior to the procedure by using the appropriate scale. It is important to recognize the patient's baseline and comfort level.

o During a moderate sedation procedure it should be in the best professional judgment of the nurse to assess for pain and address it as appropriate. The ASPMN holds the position that patients of all ages are entitled to optimal comfort during a procedure and the health care provider has the responsibility to advocate and intervene to support the best interest of the patient [8]. If pain and/or anxiety are not well controlled during the procedure, collaborate with the physician performing the procedure. Stop the procedure, evaluate the patient and seek additional support (pharmacologic, non-pharmacologic and possibly anesthesia consult).

- Some signs and symptoms of poorly controlled pain during a procedure may include but are not limited to the following:
  - Restraining patient
  - Patient is screaming, shouting, moaning, groaning or crying [8].

o Pain scales that may be used include, but are not limited to the following:

- **Numeric** [16]
  - this is the gold standard of self-reporting
  - recommended before and after procedure
- **Faces** [16]
  - Wong's faces are probably the most widely used. This scale is a self-report scale. Meaning if your patient is non-verbal and can point a finger to a face, then this may be an appropriate scale to use.
  - Recommended before or after procedure but not during for nonverbal patients.
- **Pain-AD** (Pain Assessment in Advanced Dementia) [16][17][20].

- Observational <u>(In the absence of self-report, observation of behavior is a valid approach to pain assessment)</u>.
- Used to assess pain in individuals who have dementia or other cognitive impairment and are unable to reliably communicate their pain.
- If scale has been used prior to procedure it may be sufficient enough to use during the procedure as well.

- **Behavioral Scale** [1]
  - Observational (In the absence of self-report, observation of behavior is a valid approach to pain assessment) Measures facial, activity, body movement, social, personality, mood, and physiological indicators
  - Most widely used for intubated ICU patients
  - Could potentially be utilized during a procedure.

- **Pathology Scale** (accepted in 2011 by the ASPMN) [8]
  - Patient Unable to Self-Report, but not a substitute for pain assessment.
  - Assume pain present" (APP) is shorthand for: "I have assessed this patient for pain to the extent possible given the clinical picture and the inadequacy of recognized assessment instruments in this situation. In my judgment it is reasonable to conclude that the patient is likely to be experiencing pain and I will plan my care based on that assumption" [16][17].
  - It is **only** used when all other pain assessments do not adequately quantify behaviors (i.e. chemically paralyzed patients, prior to painful procedure, patients so ill they show no behaviors)
  - Criteria for use includes: The patient has or is undergoing pathological conditions such as, a painful condition or illnesses, trauma, or surgery (non-invasive

and invasive procedures) that are likely to be painful)[17].

- Criterion for use should be documented in order to clearly explain why Pathology scale was used.
- Requires pain-relieving interventions and evaluation of effectiveness

For instance there is a patient undergoing a Percutaneous Transhepatic Cholangiogram tube placement (PTC), a painful procedure. The patient was assessed by using the numeric scale when he arrived into the procedure room. The patient scores his pain at a 4/10 in the right upper quadrant of his abdomen, which he states he has lived with for 2 weeks now and takes Oxycodone every 6hrs. Today he didn't take any medication for pain. He was given a first dose of sedation, Fentanyl and Versed as ordered, vital signs and sedation level monitored q 5min. The nurse recognizes the patient appears comfortable, eyes are closed and patient is resting quietly. The physician starts the procedure and begins telling the patient that he may feel her starting, the patient appears to be resting quietly but wakes and grimaces, clenching teeth, when the physician touches his skin to administer local anesthetic. At this point another dose of sedation is given as ordered and documentation under a behavioral scale and/ or record that the pain was caused by pathological reasons was recorded. At the completion of the procedure, when the patient is more conscious, the nurse resumes to a self report pain scale to assess the patient's pain.

Outcome Measures Tool

Every healthcare institution should have a quality and practice improvement program. This program is design to ensure best practices by reviewing and evaluating the care process and patient outcomes. This is done of course via data collection. A systematic data collection process is required at the departmental and physician level to capture important regulatory standards and any other important care process that impacts practice. The monitoring tool is one form of data collection utilized to measure the process of care and patient outcomes for moderate sedation and should be completed after every moderate sedation procedure. The tool's design should reflect all mandatory regulatory requirements. The following is the recommended documentation of process measures and patient outcomes, by The University HealthSystem Consortium (UHC) box 13 [13][19].

Box 13 **Recommended Documentation of process measures and patient outcomes, by The University HealthSystem Consortium (UHC)** [13][19].
Process Measures
Consents
NPO status
History obtained
Physical and airway patient exam completed
Anesthesia consult
Operator credentialed
Required monitoring
Patient Outcomes
Deaths
Aspirations
Reversal agents used
Unplanned admission or transfer to higher care
Cardiac/respiratory arrest

While the goals of moderate sedation includes promoting comfort and relieving anxiety for the patient, safety is by far the most critical goal of moderate sedation. Because of the possible complications associated with moderate sedation, there have been standard practice guidelines and requirements implemented by organizations and regulatory bodies to ensure patient safety and quality care. Regardless of where a moderate sedation procedure takes place in a healthcare institution, there needs to be a well organized systematic approach to ensure that the environment, personnel and documentation meet the standards of care.

Reference:

1. Ahlers, S. J. G. M., Veen, A. M. V. D., Dijk, M. V., Tibboel, D., & Knibbe, C. A. J. (2009). The use of the

behavioral pain scale to assess pain in. Anesthesia & Analgesia, doi: ANE.0b013e3181c3119e

2. The American Nurses Association, Inc. (2013). What is nursing?. Retrieved from http://www.nursingworld.org/EspeciallyForYou/What-is-Nursing

3. American Society of PeriAnesthesia Nurses. (2012-2014). *Perianesthesia nursing standards, practice recommendations and interpretive statements*. American Society of PeriAnesthesia Nurses.

4. Becker, D., & Haas, D. (2007). Management of complications during moderate and deep sedation: Respiratory and cardiovascular considerations. *Anesth Progress*, *54*(2), 59-69. Retrieved from http://www.ncbi.nlm.nih.gov/pmc/articles/PMC1893095/

5. Brent, N. J. (n.d.). When does a nurse have the right to refuse to give a patient medication? [Online forum comment]. Retrieved from Nurse.com

6. Brooke, P. S. (2009, July). Legally speaking. when can you say no? Nursing 2013, 39(7), 42-46. Retrieved from http://www.nursingcenter.com

7. Canning, P. (2007, December 29). *10 things every paramedic should know about capnography*. Retrieved from http://medicscribe.com/capnography

8. Czarnecki, M., Turner, H., Collins, P., Doellman, D., Wrona, S., & Reynolds, J. (2011). Procedural pain management: A position statement with clinical practice . doi: 1524-9042

9. Distraction Techniques for Anxiety http://www.livestrong.com/article/132949-distraction-techniques-anxiety/#ixzz2PbklAv9b

10. Education Committee of the Society of Gastroenterology Nurses and Associates, Inc. (SGNA) chaired by Trina Van Guilder, RN,BSN,CGRN. (2003). Guidelines for documentation in. Retrieved from http://www.sgna.org/Portals/0/Education/Practice Guidelines/DocumentationGuideline.pdf

11. Eslinger, M. R. (n.d.). Moderate sedation certification. Retrieved from www.sedationcertification.com
12. The joint commission. (2012). Retrieved from http://www.jointcommission.org
13. Kost, M. (2004). Moderate sedation/analgesia. (2nd ed.). St. Louis: Saunders.
14. Lazear, S. E. (2011). Moderate sedation/analgesia. Sacremento, California: CME Resource. Retrieved from http://www.netce.com/courseoverview.php?courseid=751
15. Middaugh, S. (2013). A brain for pain. John Hopkins Nursing Magazine, Retrieved from http://magazine.nursing.jhu.edu/2010/08/a-brain-for-pain/
16. Partners Against Pain. (n.d.). Pain assessment scales. Retrieved from http://www.partnersagainstpain.com/hcp/pain-assessment/tools.aspx
17. Quinn, T. (2006). Appropriate Use of "Assume Pain Present" (APP) and the Analgesic Trial in Practice and Documentation.
18. Roles & responsibilities of a nurse. (2008, April 19). Retrieved from http://nursingcrib.com/nursing-notes-reviewer/roles-responsibilities-of-a-nurse/
19. Urman, R. D, & Kaye, A. D. (2012). Moderate and deep sedation in clinical practice. New York: Cambridge University Press.
20. Warden, V, Hurley AC, Volicer, V. (2003). Development and psychometric evaluation of the Pain Assessment in Advanced Dementia (PAINAD) Scale. J Am Med Dir Assoc, 4:9-15. Developed at the New England Geriatric Research Education & Clinical Center, Bedford VAMC, MA.
21. Washington State Legislation. (n.d.). Radiologist assistant scope of practice. Retrieved from http://apps.leg.wa.gov/WAC/registerfiling.aspx?cite=246-926-300

Chapter 6

Post-Procedure

Closing the Gaps

Practice guidelines for post moderate sedation appear to be vague when compared to the PeriAnesthesia post-op nursing standards. This neglected topic leaves a bit of a gap in the delivery of care to moderately sedated patients. Some questions you may be faced with in the recovery of these patients may include:

- Can I send my patient back to their floor bed after a moderately sedated procedure or do they need to go to a phase II recovery area?
- How long does my patient need to be recovered?
- Does the procedure nurse have to escort the patient to their room with monitoring equipment?
- What is the nurse to patient ratio for patients being recovered from moderate sedation?
- Where and how long to I keep a patient who has been reversed from moderate sedation?
- What happens if my outpatient doesn't have an escort home?

Regardless of the hole in recovery (lack of guidelines) for moderately sedated patients, what the common practice boils down to is this:

> *Patients can receive sedation through a variety of methods in an operative suite or procedure room. But no matter what method was used, all patients require careful post-operative/post-procedure monitoring and assessment.*

The purpose

The purpose of post sedation monitoring is to ensure the patient achieves his/her pre-sedation level of consciousness and functioning. This period provides a time to assess, diagnose, and treat complications associated with the administration of moderate sedation. Post sedation discharge and monitoring guidelines are mandated by regulatory, accrediting, and institutional bodies to ensure patient safety and quality care. Post sedation recovery may be provided in a variety of settings, because of this, it is vital that the environment, personnel and documentation are consistent with the required practice guidelines. See box 14

Box 14	TJC
	Standards PC.13.40, PC.03 01.01,PC 03.01.07[5]

Environment
No mention of specific area only that:
- The hospital has equipment available to monitor the patient's physiological status.
- The hospital has equipment available to administer intravenous fluids and medications, and blood and blood components.
- The hospital has resuscitation equipment available.

Personnel
- A registered nurse supervises peri-operative nursing care.
- A qualified licensed independent practitioner discharges the patient from the recovery area or from the hospital. In the absence of a qualified licensed independent practitioner, patients are discharged according to criteria approved by clinical leaders.
- Patients who have received sedation or anesthesia as outpatients are discharged in the company of an individual who accepts responsibility for the patient.

Documentation
- The hospital assesses the patient's physiological status immediately after the operative or other high risk procedure and/or as the patient recovers from moderate or deep sedation or anesthesia
- The hospital monitors the patient's physiological status, mental status, and pain level at a frequency and intensity consistent with the potential effect of the operative or other high risk procedure and/or the sedation or anesthesia administered.

Environment

Post sedation monitoring may be provided in a variety of areas. Patients can be monitored in the procedure room, inpatient room, or in a post sedation recovery area. The area needs to have:

- Appropriate monitoring equipment per regulatory bodies.
- Emergency resuscitative equipment.
- And a skilled health care provider, in airway management and emergency resuscitative technique, to be present or immediately available[11].

Inpatient & Outpatient Recovery

Patients may continue to be at risk for complications even following completion of the procedure [11]. The initial 15 min after procedure is completed is the most critical period [11]. The nurse administrating the sedatives should escort the patient to a recovery area and give a bedside report to the nurse accepting patient care [7]. Patients must be transferred to a safe physical area.

The Area

The area must be appropriately equipped with monitoring devices, airway devices, crash cart and emergency equipment. Patients need to be continuously monitored in an appropriately staffed and equipped area until they return to their baseline level of consciousness and no longer at risk for cardio-respiratory complications. Within the area of recovery, their needs to be a skilled health care provider, in airway management and emergency resuscitative techniques, present or immediately available [11].

Patient transfer begins with appropriate identification, followed by report of the procedure, medications administered, complications and post procedure orders to the responsible nurse recovering patient [7][11]. Patients returning to their rooms, must have a satisfactory respiratory status and stable vital signs. A discharge scoring system ought to be used to assist in identifying those patients ready for discharge from the area where sedation took place. The Modified Aldereti Score (MAS) or the Post-

Anesthesia Discharge Score (PADSS) are two examples that can be used to identify the patients discharge readiness. A MAS of 18 < or a MAS equal to their pre-sedation baseline is acceptable for an inpatient to return to their room with recommended post procedure monitoring orders [7].

Personnel for patient returning to floor

The staffing plan (nurse to patient ratio) for patients receiving moderate sedation should reflect those guidelines from the PeriAnesthesia Nursing standards of 2012-2014. It is however, the registered nurse's prudent judgment to determine the nurse to patient ratio, patient mix, and staffing mix that reflects the patient's acuity and nursing intensity [1].

Personnel for Recovery Area

In a recovery area, the registered nurse may recover two patients or care for one recovering patient while preparing a second patient for a procedure. In addition there needs be another personnel in the recovery area in the event that a complication may arise [11]. Patients should be escorted by the procedure nurse to the recovery area. A detailed report on the procedure, medications, and other pertinent information should be communicated to the recovery nurse. The patient's vital signs (blood pressure, heart rate, respiratory rate, oxygen saturation, level of sedation, and pain) and Level of Conscious (LOC) should be monitored every 15 min for at least 30-60 min. after the administration of the last dose of moderate sedation [4][6][7][11].

Special Considerations

In the event that a patient has been reversed with the administration of reversal agents, then the patient's vital signs and level of conscious must be monitored and documented every 15 min for at least two hours following the last dose of reversal agent. If the patient is an inpatient, other than a step-down or Intensive Care Unit (ICU), then the patient must recover in the procedure suite or an appropriate post sedation recovery area. The rationale for this is re-sedation can occur within this time due to the half life of certain moderate sedations given [7][11].

Documentation

Post procedure recovery documentation should include:

- The patient's physiological status. Generally this is VS and LOC every 15 mins until patient meets discharge status from sedation area or to home.

- A post anesthesia scoring system a such as the Alderte should be used and documented. Scoring systems are a good indicator to determine the patient's discharge status.

- Education on discharge instructions pertaining to procedure and sedation. This is provided to the floor nurse receiving the patient or to a responsible adult escorting patient home.

Discharge to home

For outpatients being discharged to home post procedure they need to meet the following criteria [4][5][6][7]:

- Discharged by a qualified licensed independent practitioner
.
- Patients should meet there pre-sedation baseline and discharge scoring system score.
- The patient meets baseline verbal communication (talking).
- The patient is easily arousable and protective reflexes are intact.
- Fluid intake: Not all patients have to tolerate fluids before discharge. Guidelines now only require that certain populations, such as diabetics achieve this function.
- Voiding: generally this only includes those patients that have had a peri-operative urinary catheterization, pelvic, genitourinary, rectal surgery or procedures, or who have had a history of urinary retention. Those patients that do not void prior to discharge need to be sent home with clear instructions seeking medical attention if they do not void for a period of eight hours after discharge.
- Documentation concerning the discharge status of the patient must be present.

- Patient being discharged to home must have a safe transportation prearranged with a responsible adult, prior to the procedure by the patient per TJC, AAAHC, ASA, and SGNA standards.
  - According to the Society of Peri-anesthesia Nurses Standards or Perianesthesia Nursing, **a responsible person** is someone who is physically and mentally able to make decisions for the patient's welfare if necessary. This person must understand and comply with post anesthetic care instructions [1].
    - The responsible person needs to be 18 yrs and older.
    - A taxi driver or bus driver is not considered a responsible person. *AMA*
  - Patients should not receive any anesthesia or sedation and then drive home. Driving after receiving sedation is not considered safe. It is the obligation of the caregiver to cancel the case, arrange transportation, or admit the patient. As a part of ensuring patient safety and providing best care, healthcare institutions, need to implement policies that aim to avoid discharge without an escort [2].

Approaches to transportation and responsible person issues.

Some patients simply do not have someone to escort them home, let alone watch them. Here are a few strategies to consider:
- Address the importance of having an adult escort drive or escort the patient home during the pre-procedure clinic visit or phone evaluations.
- The healthcare institution's sedation committee should come up with a plan with the social worker to develop a list of alternatives for patients who do not have a responsible adult to help them.
  - Such alternatives may include:
    - A list of transportation resources such as church volunteers, van services, homeless shelters, and patient medical escorts.

- Offer a "hotel bed" where a patient can stay for a small fee in a hospital setting overnight, without nursing care but emergency access.
- Prepare a list of volunteers within the community willing to stay with the patient and drive them home.

Discharge instructions

Post procedural instructions should be provided to the patient and the responsible caregiver. These instructions should address the following:

- Diet
- Level of activity
    - Do not drive, operate equipment, consume alcoholic beverages, and make important personal or business decisions for 24hrs [6][7].
- Wound/ dressing care
    - Address fever, bleeding, dressing changes, pain and discomfort.
- Prescription drug education
    - Avoid taking any hypnotics, sedatives, muscle relaxants, narcotics unless prescribed and consulted with your physician[6].
- Follow up appointment
- Emergency contact number
    - For physician or after hours emergency centers

There should also be documentation that both the patient and responsible adult signs regarding understanding of the post sedation instructions before discharge. There should also be a signed verification that the patient will be accompanied home by a responsible person[7][11].

Lastly, a well organized healthcare institution needs to provide a follow up phone call 24 hrs post discharge to obtain any incidence of complications related to the procedure, sedation, pain, instructions, and patient satisfaction [7].

References:

1. American Society of PeriAnestheisa Nursing. (2012, November). Frequently asked question, responsible adult. Retrieved from http://www.aspan.org/ClinicalPractice/FAQs/tabid/14107/Default.aspx
2. (n.d.). Car accidents after ambulatory surgery in patients without escort. Retrieved from http'/methodistanesthesia.com/articles/article_19.pdf
3. (n.d.). Current opinion in anesthesiology. (2009). Ambulatory anesthesia, 22(6), 748-754. doi: 10.1097/aco.0b013e328331d498
4. Eslinger, M. R. (n.d.). Moderate sedation certification. Retrieved from www.sedationcertification.com
5. The joint commission. (2012). Retrieved from http://www.jointcommission.org
6. Kost, M. (2004). Moderate sedation/analgesia. (2nd ed.). St. Louis: Saunders.
7. Lazear, S. E. (2011). Moderate sedation/analgesia. Sacremento, California: CME Resource. Retrieved from http://www.netce.com/courseoverview.php?courseid=751
8. Partners Against Pain. (n.d.). Pain assessment scales. Retrieved from http://www.partnersagainstpain.com/hcp/pain-assessment/tools.aspx
9. Quinn, T. (2006). Appropriate Use of "Assume Pain Present" (APP) and the Analgesic Trial in Practice and Documentation.
10. Roles & responsibilities of a nurse. (2008, April 19). Retrieved from http://nursingcrib.com/nursing-notes-reviewer/roles-responsibilities-of-a-nurse/
11. Urman, R. D, & Kaye, A. D. (2012). Moderate and deep sedation in clinical practice. New York: Cambridge University Press.

Chapter 7

Medications

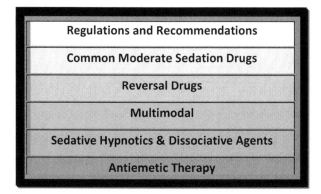

Regulations and Recommendations

Each state in the U.S has different regulations regarding who may administer sedation and what medications can be administered. One must be sure to check with their state board of nursing to see what medications they are eligible to administer. For instance a nurse in WV can manage a paralytic or propofol drip in an intubated patient and can also administer ketamine for a patient on palliative care, but according to the state board of nursing that same nurse cannot administer paralytics, propofol, and/or ketamine for moderate sedation purposes.

In the following three boxes are some regulations on the administration of moderate sedation by TJC as well as recommendations from the American Nurses Association, the American Society of Anesthesiologists Task Force on Sedation, and Analgesia by Non-Anesthesiologists.

> **TJC Standard PC.13.20** [20]
>
> Individuals administering moderate sedation are qualified and have appropriate credentials to manage patients at whatever level of sedation or anesthesia is achieved, either intentionally or unintentionally.

American Society of Anesthesiologists Task Force on Sedation and Analgesia by Non-Anesthesiologists Recommendations [20]

The individuals responsible for the patient receiving moderate sedation/analgesia should understand the pharmacology of the medications being administered, as well as the antagonist for opioids and benzodiazepines.

The combination of analgesic and sedatives may be given as appropriate for the procedure being performed.

Intravenous sedatives and analgesics should be given in small incremental doses. Sufficient amount if time should be given between doses to allow for each dose to take effect.

Even though moderate sedation may be intended while using propofol or methohexial than requirements for deep sedation should be followed.

Reversal agents for benzodiazepines and opioids should be available.

The American Nurses Association [20]

The registered nurse managing the care of the patient receiving IV moderate sedation is able to:
- Anticipate and recognize potential complications related to moderate sedation.
- Posses the required knowledge and skills to assess, diagnose, and intervene in the event of a negative outcome per institutional policies and procedures.
- Demonstrate airway management and resuscitation
- Demonstrate knowledge of legal ramifications associated with moderate sedation, including the nurse's liabilities and responsibilities.

A failure to understand the clinical effects of each medication administered, especially when used in combinations, could result in an increase in patient mortality.

Common Moderate Sedation Drugs

There are many different types of medications that can be used for moderate sedation. However, it is ultimately up to the state and institution on which types of medications you are allowed to administer under a credential LIP.

Presently, an opioid and benzodiazepine combination appears to be the most common and preferable choice for a nurse and physician team. Although commonly used, the action of these medications together increases the risk of oxygen desaturation and cardiorespiratory complications. Because of this, it is always good to keep reversal agents for opiates and benzodiazepines readily available.

There are other medications that can be used for procedural sedation which are gaining popularity for their minimal hemodynamic effects. Other popular sedative choices include propofol, ketamine, and precedex. In addition etomidate and nitrous oxide seem to be emerging in literature for procedural sedation [27][37].

Because moderate sedation administration by a LIP and nurse team occur quite frequently for many types of patients and procedures, it is imperative that these teams fully understand the risks associated with each class of medications commonly used for moderate sedation. The next following paragraphs briefly summarize common classes used for moderate sedation and considerations to keep in mind.

Benzodiazepines [9][20][21][37]

Benzodiazepines are highly lipid soluble and rapidity enters the central nervous system. Their amnesic, anxiolytic and sedatives properties make them well suited for moderate sedation. Their minimal cardiovascular and respiratory effects in healthy patients also make them a conservative drug of choice for most procedural sedation. Even though benzodiazepines effects on the respiratory system may be minimal they still decrease upper airway muscle tone and depress the hypoxemic drive causing hypoventilation. Patients that tend to be affected the most by these actions include those who have OSA, COPD, difficult airways, liver and/or renal disease. Other patients that must be administered benzodiazepines cautiously are the elderly and those who are pregnant. The elderly, especially should not be given long acting benzodiazepines due to their decreased protein stores. This is important because benzodiazepines are 97-98% protein bound and the effects of action are potentiated in this population, leading to excessive sedation, cognitive impairment and even falls.

Benzodiazepines should be administered at recommended doses and with careful titration. Large doses of benzodiazepines can lower b/p accompanied by a response in heart rate. It's important to remember that benzodiazepines at even small doses can increase the actions of many drugs. Some drugs commonly affected by this class include:

- H-2 blocking drugs such as cimetidine (Tagamet) or ranitidine (Zantac) which can also lead to benzodiazepine overdose.
- metoprolol, propranolol, and digitalis can be potentiated by benzodiazepines causing the development of symptomatic Bradycardia.

Benzodiazepines are not usually administered alone to provide moderate sedation. They are often given in combination with an opioid which potentiates the effects of benzodiazepines. Keep in mind that even though this synergistic effect is sought after, it can cause serious respiratory depression. Some common benzodiazepines used for moderate sedation are diazepam, midazolam, and Lorazepam

Diazepam (Valium)

In the 1960's, Valium was developed by the Swiss pharmaceutical giant Hoffmann-La Roche and approved for use in 1963. Valium was first used by psychiatrists for the short-term treatment of anxiety. Today Valium is still used to treat short term anxiety for visits to the dentist, MRI and other short procedures. It is also mostly is used by neurologists for treating certain types of epilepsy and spastic activity [33][34].

Valium is given via PO, IV, or rectally. The PO forms probably the most common form of administration. Its length of action is approximately 1 to 8 hours. However, its half-life can vary from 20 to 50 hours in a healthy adult.

Considerations in the administration of Valium [8][9][29]:

- The dose administration for the elderly, neonates, and those with severe hepatic disorders, should be reduced due to their risk for prolongation of action.
- When given IV burns at insertion site.
- Diazepam in late pregnancy, especially high doses, may result in <u>floppy infant syndrome</u> [16].

Diazepam (Valium) [29]			
Route	Onset	Peak	Duration
IV	1-5 min	10 min	2-4 hrs
PO	15-60 min	60 min	3-6 hrs

Valium Titration Recommendation [29]		
Population	Dose over 2 min	MAX Dose
Adult	1-2 mg	10-20mg in 60 min
Geriatric		
Pulm & Hepatic Impairment		
Pediatric	0.1-0.3mg/kg	

Potential Adverse Reactions [29]

Phlebitis at site of injection	Hiccups	Diplopia
Bradycardia	Apnea	Urticaria
Hypotension	Confusion	Agitation
Respiratory depression	Rash	

Midazolam (Versed) [20][21][37]

Versed was also developed by Hoffmann-La Roche in the 1970s. This benzodiazepine has a rapid onset and short acting action that can be given via oral, rectal, Intra-venous, intramuscular, and intranasally (off label use, usually for peds). It is a water soluble drug making it less painful to administer IV as opposed to Ativan or Valium. Versed is 2-3 times more potent than valium and its anterograde amnesic effects are stronger than its sedative effect. Versed's various characteristics makes it the most favorable in its class.

Considerations for administering Versed [20][21][37]:

- Not to be used in patients with acute narrow angle glaucoma and shock.
- May prolong bleeding times in patients who are on Heparin.
- Half-life may double in the elderly due to decreases in age related hepatic flow and enzyme activity.
- Caution should be taken when used in the morbidly obese due to their volume of distribution.
- Versed can cause or increase coughing.

Midazolam (Versed) [8][29]			
Route	Onset	Peak	Duration
IV	1-5 min	3-5 min	15min-6 hrs
IM	5-15 min	15-60 min	2-6 hrs
PO	10 min or less	30 min	2-6hrs

Versed Titration Recommendation [8][29]		
Population	Dose over 2 min	Max Dose
Adult	0.5mg-2mg	3.0 mg can titrate higher
Geriatric	0.25mg-0.5mg	2.0 mg
Pulm & Hepatic Impairment	0.25mg-0.5mg	2.0 mg
Pediatric	0.025mg/kg	0.1 mg/kg

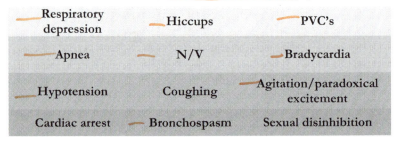

Potential Adverse Reactions [8][29]

Respiratory depression	Hiccups	PVC's
Apnea	N/V	Bradycardia
Hypotension	Coughing	Agitation/paradoxical excitement
Cardiac arrest	Bronchospasm	Sexual disinhibition

Ativan

Ativan is most known for its use in anxiety symptoms. It was first introduced in 1977, at this time it was also approved by U.S. Food and Drug Administration as an effective oral anxiolytic in anxiety symptoms. Ativan is an intermediate acting benzodiazepine that has double the potency of versed and a poor metabolite activity. Its length of action ranges from 6-8hours. This benzodiazepine is frequently used for prolong sedation and most often it is seen in the intensive care unit [27].

Considerations for administering Ativan [2][29]:

- Contraindicated in patients with acute narrow-angle glaucoma
- Contraindicated in patients with sleep apnea syndrome and with severe respiratory insufficiency.

Lorazepam(Ativan)[2][29]			
Route	Onset	Peak	Duration
IV	5-20 min	up to 2 hrs	6-8hrs
IM	20-30 min	up to 2 hrs	6-8hrs
PO	15-60 min	1-6 hrs	8-12hrs

Ativan Titration Recommendation [2][29]

Population	Dose over 2 min	MAX Dose
Adult	0.05mg/kg	2 mg IV or 4mg IM
Geriatric	Not recommended	
Pulm & Hepatic Impairment		
Pediatric	0.02-0.09mg/kg	

Potential Adverse Reactions [2][29]

Confusion	Drowsiness, dizziness, tiredness
Depressed mood, thoughts of suicide or hurting yourself	Blurred vision
Hyperactivity, agitation, hostility	Sleep problems
Feeling light-headed, fainting	Hallucinations

Opioids (Narcotics) [9][20][21][37]

Opioids are potent analgesics that when used in combination with benzodiazepines provide adequate moderate sedation for potentially painful procedures. Some common opioid agonists used in moderate sedation are Fentanyl, Morphine, Dilaudid, and Demerol. Opioids bind to mu, kappa, delta and sigma receptors in the central nervous system, varying perception and emotional response to pain. They can produce sedation alone, respiratory depression, and at high doses will produce a diminished level of consciousness.

The most common side effects associated with opioids, with the exception of Demerol, is bradycardia and hypotension. Although not as profound as benzodiazepines, opioids do cause respiratory depression. As doses increase so does the risk of cardiovascular and respiratory complications. Opioids that release histamines such as morphine and meperidine, have a greater affect on the respiratory system, especially those with a history of asthma. Other side effects to consider are nausea and vomiting. Opioids tend to stimulate the vomiting center in the brain which causes nausea after the administration of these medications. The last side effect to keep in mind is the use of opioids in neurologically compromised patients. This is due to opioids ability to increase in intracranial via increasing the cerebral blood flow and metabolic rate.

Box 15	Hierarchy of Potency
	100mcg Fentanyl IV is equivalent to:
	1.5 mg of Dilaudid IV
	7.5 mg of Methadone PO
	30 mg of Morphine PO
	75 mg of Demerol
	Reference: http://www.globalrph.com/narcotic.cgi

Fentanyl Citrate (Sublimaze)

Fentanyl was first created in 1959 by Paul Janssen under the newly formed Janssen Pharmaceutical Company. In the 1960s, Sublimaze was its trade name and it was introduced as an intravenous anesthetic [12]. Fentanyl is the favorable choice when used in moderate sedation due to its low histamine release, low emetic activity, rapid onset, and short duration of action. This opioid compared to other opioids in its class, also has minimal cardiovascular depressive effects [27][32].

Considerations when administering Fentanyl [8][21][29][32]:

- Alterations in respiratory rate and alveolar ventilation can occur. As the dose of Fentanyl increases the respiratory depression does as well. Because every drug affects every person differently, a small dose of Fentanyl can cause apnea.

- Narcan and Atropine are two drugs that should be readily available during moderate sedation procedures. Narcan is the reversal for Fentanyl's side effects and Atropine counteracts any severe and symptomatic bradycardia.

- The recommended dose for the geriatric population should be reduced by 50% or more.
- Should be used with caution in patients with compromised airway and ventilation such as those with COPD.
- Should be used with caution in patients who are bradycardiac.
- Should be used with caution in patients with liver and renal disease.
- Fentanyl's respiratory depressant effects generally last longer than its pain relieving effects.
- Do not mix with barbiturates
- Fentanyl can cause chest wall rigidity which is rare, but can be life threatening. These patients will not be able to be ventilated. Successful resuscitation includes the administration of succinylcholine by anesthesia personal and Naloxone (Narcan) should be administered as well.
-

Fentanyl Citrate (Sublimaze) [8][9][29]

Route	Onset	Peak	Duration
IV	1 min or less	5-15 min	30-60 min
IM	5-8 min	15-20 min	1-2 hrs
PO	5-15 min	20-30 min	1-2 hrs

Fentanyl Titration Recommendation [8][9][29]

Population	Dose over 2 min	Max Dose
Adult	25-100 mcg	200mcg
Geriatric	12.5-50 mcg	
Pulm & Hepatic Impairment	12.5-50 mcg	
Pediatric	0.5-2mcg/kg	

Potential Adverse Reactions [8][9][29]

Chest wall rigidity, rare, but can occur with rapid administration	Agitation
Respiratory depression, apnea	Increased ICP
N/V Delays gastric emptying	Hypotension
Biliary tract spasms	Bradycardia
Euphoria	Constipation

Hydromorphone Hydrochloride (Dilaudid)

Hydromorphone was first created and researched in Germany in 1924; it was introduced to the market in 1926 under the brand name Dilaudid [11]. Dilaudid is derivative of morphine with 5 to 6 times the potency of morphine. However unlike morphine it results in less histamine release, making it a good alternative to Fentanyl if needed [37]. Lower risks of excessive sedation or respiratory depression occur in Dilaudid in comparison with other opioids of its class.

Considerations when administrating Dilaudid [20][21][29] :

- Narcan (Naloxone) is the reversal.
- Reduce dose by 50% when administrating to elderly patients.
- Contraindicated in neuro patients, Increases intra-cranial pressure.
- Respiratory depression is dose dependent.
- Due to its long onset, peak and duration some physicians like to use it in addition with Fentanyl & Versed for procedures such as bone biopsies.

Hydromorphone Hydrochloride (Dilaudid) [8][29]

Route	Onset	Peak	Duration
IV	1-15 min	0.25-1 hr	2-3 hrs
IM	15 min	0.5-1hr	4-5 hrs
PO	30 min	1.5-2 hrs	4 hrs

Hydromorphone Hydrochloride (Dilaudid) [8][29]

Population	Dose over 2-3 min	Max Dose
Adult	0.1-0.4mg q 5-15 min	2-4mg hr
Geriatric	reduce dose by 50%	
Renal & Hepatic Impairment	1-2 mg q 4-6 hrs	
Pediatric	0.015 mg/kg slow IV/IM/PR/SC q4-6hr PRN	

Potential Adverse Reactions [8][29]

Cardiac arrest
MI
QT-interval prolongation
Severe cardiac arrhythmias
ST segment elevation
Syncope ventricular tachycardia
Angina pectoris
Bradycardia

Agitation
Dizziness
Euphoria
Sedation
Seizures
Visual disturbances
Weakness

Anticholinergic effects:
Dry mouth
Palpitation
Tachycardia
Urinary retention

Biliary tract spasm
(sphincter of Odes)

Respiratory arrest

Constipation, Nausea, Vomiting

Hypotension

Increased ICP

Morphine Sulfate

Morphine is an analgesic for pain that is generally reserved for the relief of moderate to severe acute and chronic pain. This medication is normally seen being utilized for post-surgical pain relief in the PACU and acute traumatic pain in the ED, as well as the treatment for myocardial infarctions or angina. Morphine can also be used in moderate sedation as well, but is not as popular as its counter partners. Morphine has the appealing feature of a rapid onset but its action of releasing histamine, causing unwanted side effects, makes it less popular than Fentanyl or Dilaudid.

A form of morphine can be dated back as far as the byzantine times (330-1453). The city of Byzantine later became Constantinople. In December of 1804 in Paderborn, Friedrich Sertürner discovered morphine as the first active alkaloid extracted from the opium poppy plant. Serturner named morphine after Morpheus, the Greek god of dreams, for its tendency to cause sleep [3]. Sertürner and Company first marketed morphine to the general public in 1817 as an analgesic and as a treatment for opium and alcohol addiction. During the American Civil War it became known that morphine was more addicting than alcohol or opium. The extensive use during the war led to approximately 400,000 soldiers suffering from "soldiers disease" aka morphine addiction. The public however believed it to be just a fabrication. In 1914 Morphine became a controlled substance in the US under the Harrison Narcotics Tax Act. Morphine was the most commonly abused narcotic analgesic in the world until heroin was synthesized and came into use [4][13][23].

Morphine Sulfate (MSO4) [8][29]			
Route	Onset	Peak	Duration
IV	1 min or less	5-20 min	4-7 hrs
IM	5-10 min	30-60 min	4-7 hrs
PO	1 hr or less	1-2 hrs	6-12 hrs

MSO4 Titration Recommendation [8][29]		
Population	Dose every 15min	Max Dose
Adult	2-10 mg	10mg in 60 min
Geriatric	Decreased doses	
Renal & Hepatic Impairment	Decreased doses	
Pediatric	0.05-0.1mg/kg	

Potential Adverse Reactions [8][29]

Bradycardia, arrhythmias	Somnolence, euphoria
Chest wall rigidity	Constipation
Respiratory depression Bronchospasms laryngospasms	Nausea, Vomiting
Hypotension	Biliary tract spasm (sphincter of Odes)

Narcan (Naloxone) is the reversal

Considerations for the administration of Morphine [8][29]:

- Histamine release action affects the respiratory system. It depresses respiratory volume and rate. Therefore the use of morphine in patients with respiratory diseases should be used with caution. Have airway equipment and Narcan readily available.

- Should be avoided in patients with bronchial asthma.

- Elderly have an increased risk of respiratory depression.

- Histamine release action leads to decrease in systemic vascular resistance causing high risk for hypotension. Have IV bolus available if needed.

- Should be avoided in patients suspected of having paralytic ileus.

- Should be used with caution in patients with convulsive disorders and may induce seizures

- Morphine has the potential to elevate CSF pressure and therefore should be used with caution for patients with head injuries, lesions or preexisting increased intracranial pressure (ICP).

- May be beneficial to use in moderately sedating a patient with a persistent and continuous cough. Morphine depresses cough reflex by direct effect on the cough center in the medulla. *codeine?*

Meperidine Hydrochloride (Demerol)

Meperidine, aka Demerol, is an analgesic that affects the central nervous systems and smooth muscle organs. The primary use for Meperidine is reserved for relief of moderate to severe pain, preoperatively, and for moderate sedation[29]. It is also thought that Meperidine is superior in treating pain associated with biliary spasm or renal colic due to its antispasmodic effects, however this may controversial. Meperidine is similar to morphine as in that is too has an action to release histamines. It is however less potent than morphine (8-10 mg of Meperdine is approximately equivalent to 1 mg of morphine)[20].

Meperidine was first created in 1930's in anticipation of generating a superior anticholinergic/ anti-spasmodic agent. Otto Schaumann of Germany, first recognized its analgesic properties [23]. Shortly after this discovery, scientists and pharmacologists began using meperidine to treat chronic pain. Thus began the long process of marketing a potent new pain killer [15].

Meperidine Hydrochloride (Demerol) [8][29]			
Route	Onset	Peak	Duration
IV	1 min	5-20 min	2-4 hrs
IM	1-5 min	30-50 min	2-4 hrs
PO	15-45 min	60 min	2-4hrs

Demerol Titration Recommendation [8][29]		
Population	Dose	Max Dose
Adult	25mg	100mg in 60 min
Geriatric	< 25mg	
Renal & Hepatic Impairment	<25mg	
Pediatric	1-1.5mg/kg	100 mg

Potential Adverse Reactions [8][29]

Bradycardia, Palpations, Shock, Cardiac arrest, Tachycardia	Sedation, Euphoria, Weakness
Agitation, Disorientation, Hallucinations, Tremors	Constipation
Severe Respiratory Depression Arrest Use in caution with COPD or hypoxic patients	Nausea/Vomiting
Orthostatic Hypotension	Biliary tract spasm (sphincter of Odes)

Narcan (Naloxone) is the reversal

Considerations for the administration of Meperidine [20][21][29]:

- Histamine release action affects the respiratory system. It depresses respiratory volume and rate. Therefore the use of meperidine in patients with respiratory diseases should be used with caution. Have airway equipment and Narcan readily available.
- Should be avoided in patients with bronchial asthma.
- Elderly have an increased risk of respiratory depression.
- Histamine release action leads to decrease in systemic vascular resistance causing high risk for hypotension. Have IV bolus available if needed.
- Should be avoided in patients suspected of having paralytic ileus.

- Should be used with caution in patients with convulsive disorders and may induce seizures
- Meperidine has the potential to elevate CSF pressure and therefore should be used with caution for patients with head injuries, lesions or preexisting increased intracranial pressure (ICP).
- May be beneficial to use in moderately sedating a patient with a persistent and continuous cough. Meperidine may depress cough reflex by direct effect on the cough center in the medulla more effectively than morphine.

Reversals/Antagonists [9][20][21][32]

If the patients pre procedure assessment, past medical history and labs has been reviewed, along with appropriate titration of moderate sedation during the procedure, then reversal agents should not be needed. However, if it is needed, the advantage of antagonists is they can be titrated slowly to reverse deep sedation and respiratory depression, without compromising sedative effects. This allows continuation of the patient's procedure under moderate sedation. Keep in mind slow titration may not be an option if severe cardiopulmonary complications occur.

Flumazenil and Naloxone are the two reversals for benzodiazepines and opioids. Both Flumazenil and Naloxone will reverse the pharmacologic effects of medication that react on the receptors of the Central Nervous System (CNS). However, their length of action is generally short and maybe needed repeated doses. The goal of reversing moderate sedation is to arouse the patient from an unintentional sedation level that is no longer within your ability to manage safely. By no means should the patient be reversed simply because the LIP wants the patient to recover faster.

In the event that a patient has been reversed with the administration of reversal agents, then the patient must be monitored (vital signs and level of conscious) every 15 min. for at least two hours following the last dose of reversal agent. If the patient is an inpatient, other than in the step-down or Intensive Care Unit (ICU), then the patient must recover in the procedure suite or an appropriate post sedation recovery area. The rationale for this is re-sedation can occur within this time due to the half-life of certain moderate sedations given.

Flumazenil (Romazicon)

Flumazenil is a benzodiazepine antagonist. It can be used to fully or partial reverse benzodiazepine overdose.

Reversal for Benzodiazepines: Flumazenil (Romazicon) [8][29]					
Route	Onset	Peak	Duration	Dose	Max
IV bolus	1-3 min	6-10 min	45-90 min	0.2mg over 15 sec to 1 min Peds: 0.01mg/kg over 15 sec	repeat dose every 1 min until 1mg.

Special considerations in the administration of Flumazenil
[8][9][20][21][29]:

- The manufacturers of Flumazenil do not recommend the use for patients under the age of 18. However, it is safe and effective to give an individualized dosage to children between the ages 1-17. The use of Flumazenil safety and effectiveness have not been established for the use if re-sedation occurs. Children ages 1-5 are more adapt to experience re-sedation.
- When giving Flumazenil, it should be given in 0.2mg increments every 1 min for a max dose of 1 mg.
- Patient response generally occurs within 3 minutes after administration.
- If response to medication after 3 minutes does not occur, a code response team should be notified immediately.

- Patients that have been dependent on benzodiazepine for long periods of time can experience seizure activity when reversed by Flumazenil.
- Agitation, anxiety and convulsions may occur if patients receive an over dose of Flumazenil.
- Flumazenil has a short duration and re-sedation can occur, because of this it is best that patients be monitored in a recovery, step-down or ICU like environment for 120 minutes.

Potential Adverse Reactions [8][29]

Re-sedation once drug has worn off	Headache
Sweating & flushing	Blurred vision
Bradycardia, Tachycardia, Dysthymias	Confusion, Convulsions

Naloxone Hydrochloride (Narcan)

Narcan was developed by Sankyo in the 1960s (as per US Patent 3254088 - Morphine Derivative). It is used as a complete or partial reversal of opioid depression, respiratory and cardiovascular depression caused by opioids [29].

Narcan reverses

Respiratory depression

Hypotension

Hypercapnia

Sedation

euphoria associated with the

administration of opioids [9].

Special considerations [8][9][29]:

- Titrate slowly to desired effect. Complete reversal will produce total reversal of analgesia.
- Complete reversal may cause procedure hypertension, excitation, and tachycardia. Some instances patient may set up on procedure table quickly.

- If given rapidly, non-cardiogenic pulmonary edema may occur.
- If no response occurs after 2mg, code team should be notified immediately.
- Monitor the patient closely in the post procedure for approximately 90-120 minutes, for possibility of re-sedation. Narcan has a shorter duration than most opioids.

If the initial sedative/narcotic is properly titrated to effect, reversal should not be needed. However, if it is needed, usually small doses are adequate. The larger doses found in resources are indicated for significant overdoses as seen in obtunded/comatose patients [9].

Reversal for Narcotics: Naloxone Hydrochloride (Narcan) Dosage [8][29]		
	Dose	Max
Adult	0.04mg	repeat dose every 2-3 min until 2 mg if needed
Peds	0.01 mg or 0.1 mg/kg	repeat dose every 2-3 min until 0.2mg/kg if needed

Reversal for Narcotics: Naloxone Hydrochloride (Narcan) [8][29]				
	Route	Onset	Peak	Duration
Adult	IV bolus or infusion	1-2 min	5-15 min	1-4 hrs
Peds	IV bolus or infusion	1-2 min	5-15 min	1-4 hrs

Potential Adverse Reactions [8][29]

Pulmonary edema	Tremors
Hypertension	Seizures
Tachycardia, arrhythmias, V-tach, V-fib	Excitement

Multi-Modal Therapy

A multimodal approach involves having several modes or modalities of medications to control pain and sometimes anxiety. The rationale for this strategy is centered on the synergistic effects between different classes of medications. With any procedure or surgery the most important step is to assure the patient that any pain is going to be controlled. Patients who enter the hospital generally anticipate a painful procedure and magnify any pain and anxiety they may feel. Not only does the patients experience sensitivity to pain and anxiety, but their complex procedure may also complicate the ability to control these symptoms . A multi-modal therapy for pain and anxiety may be something to consider in this population and for more complex procedures.

Pain

The multimodal approach has long been endorsed by many professional organizations, such as the American Society of Anesthesiologists (ASA), American Pain Society and the American Society for Pain Management Nursing [28]. The rationale for this strategy is centered on the synergistic effects between different classes of analgesics. This method also allows both individual opioids to potentially be reduced, lowering the incidence of adverse outcomes, and the prevention of pain before it starts [28].

While there is no particular "gold standard" multimodal regimen to use pre, intra, or post procedure, Acetaminophen and Ketorolac appear to be common adjuncts to opioids in controlling pain intra and post procedure [30].

Acetaminophen (Ofirmev IV)

The IV form of Acetaminophen was approved by the U.S in November, 2010, for the use of mild to moderate pain and moderate to severe pain with adjunctive opioid analgesics [22]. Acetaminophen inhibits prostaglandins that may provide as mediators of pain and fever in the CNS. Since it's release in IV form, it has been proven to be an effective pain controlling medication when given with opioids. In fact it's administration before and during surgeries have proven to be very beneficial in the amount of pain experienced by the patient after the procedure. It has also help prevent the use of rescue mediations and adverse reactions from excessive opioid use.

Studies

Acetaminophen multimodal approach, has been successively utilized in surgical cases. In 22 studies involving patients undergoing surgery, 10 of the 14 studies reported less opioid consumption, and a lower percentage of requiring rescue medications. The studies concluded that IV acetaminophen effective as an analgesic agent across a range of surgical procedures [28].

During another study involving 82 patients undergoing a total abdominal hysterectomy, patients were randomized into 3 groups. The first group received IV acetaminophen before surgery, the 2nd group received IV acetaminophen at closure, and the 3rd group was the placebo. The conclusion included both IV acetaminophen groups required significantly lower morphine administration than the placebo group. The 1st group also received less morphine consumption than the 2nd IV acetaminophen group. Overall the 1st group had both lower incidences of adverse effects and the shortest hospital stay [28].

Special Considerations of Acetaminophen [1][8][29]

- Beneficial over oral or rectal due to its avoidance of first pass metabolism. Exposes liver to 50% less acetaminophen when compared to oral route at the same dose.
- If given higher than recommended can cause may result in hepatic injury.
- Acetaminophen drug/substance interactions to keep in mind include:
    - Warfarin, Plavix and thrombolytic agents (increases bleeding)

- Alcohol, barbiturates, tegretol, dilantin, and CYP2E1 inducers/inhibitors.
- Aspirin decrease acetaminophen effects.
  - Decreases the effectiveness of diuretics or antihypertensives.
- Once opened use within 6 hrs.
- Safety not established in patients <2 yrs old.
- Should not be given in patients with severe hepatic impairment or active liver disease.
- Avoid in pregnancy, give only if needed.

Acetaminophen (Ofirmev IV) [1][22]

Onset	Peak	Duration	Max	Direction
15min	1 hr	4-6 hr	4g per day for adults and children weighing >50kg	Infuse over 15 min. Once opened use within 6 hr.

Potential Adverse Effects [22]

Anxiety	Hypertension/ Hypotension	Muscle spasms
Atelectasis	Elevated Liver enzymes	Hypokalemia

Ketorolac (Toradol)

Toradol was discovered in 1989 by Syntex Corp and approved by FDA on 30 November of the same year [18][36]. Toradol is a short term nonsteroidal anti-inflammatory (NSAIDs) pain medication that acts by decreasing hormones the cause of inflammation and pain in the body [18]. This NSAID is a popular medication in the treatment of moderate to severe pain, especially when given as an adjunct to opioids for post surgical pain [6].

Studies

There are many studies proving the significance in Toradol's opioid sparing effects when given pre-operatively.

One study used intravenous 30 mg ketorolac as a preemptive analgesic for patients undergoing ankle fracture repair. The conclusion indicated fewer patients experienced pain and nausea in post surgical nausea if given Toradol preemptively [25].

Another study using ketorolac preemptive for postoperative third molar surgical pain, showed similar results. Throughout the 12 hr investigation period, patients reported having significantly lower pain scores in the ketorolac pretreated sides when compared with the post-treated sides. Patients also experienced a lesser postoperative analgesic consumption and a considerably longer time before rescue analgesic were used [26].

Considerations in the administration of Toradol [18][19][29]:

- Like any other NSAID, this medication can increase your risk of life-threatening heart or circulation problems, including heart attack or stroke. Risks are increased the longer it is used.
- Should not be administered for more than 5 days or 20 doses.
- Should not be given to patients who have:
    - severe kidney disease
    - a bleeding or blood clotting disorder
    - a closed head injury or bleeding in your brain
    - a stomach ulcer or a history of stomach or intestinal bleeding
- This medication should not be used in during pregnancy or patients who are breast feeding, may be harmful to an unborn baby. It is listed as FDA pregnancy category C in first and 2nd trimester and a category D in the 3rd trimester of pregnancy.
- **CONTRAINDICATED for the treatment of perioperative pain in the setting of coronary artery bypass graft (CABG) surgery.**
- Toradol can not significantly be cleared from the blood stream by dialysis.

- In patients with moderately elevated serum creatinine, ketorolac injection should not exceed 60 mg per day.

Ketorolac (Toradol) Dosage [18][19][29]		
	Dose	**Half-life**
Adult IV	30mg every 6 hr Max dose 120mg/day	5.6 hr average
Geriatric IV	<50kg=<60mg per day for	5-7hr
Pediatric IV 2-16 yrs	1mg/kg Max dose = 30mg a day Or 0.5mg/kg/day Max dose=15mg	1.6 – 5.8 hr
Renal Insufficiency		6 and 19 hours
Hepatic Insufficiency		No real difference from healthy adult

Ketorolac (Toradol) [18][19][29]			
	Onset	**Peak**	**Duration**
Adult IV	10min	1-2 hr	6hr

Most Common Side Effects [18][19][29]

Swelling of face, fingers, lower legs, ankles, and/or feet	Sores, ulcers, or white spots on lips or in mouth
Bruising	Skin rash or itching

Sedation Adjuncts

Benadryl (diphenhydramine)

Chemist George Rieveschi, in the 1940s, first discovered histamine receptors while researching potential muscle relaxers. What he noticed was specific histamine receptors could be controlled by medications, hence his development of Benadryl [38]. Benadryl is an antihistamine with anticholinergic and sedative effects used to treat allergy symptoms, suppress coughs, induce sleep, and motion sickness [9].

Antihistamines like Benadryl can cause sedation but they are less effective than benzodiazepines. For this reason they are not primarily used as a anxiolytic or sedative. They can however, be a beneficial adjunct in potentiating sedation when benzodiazepines are ineffective alone. Antihistamines also have a antiemetic property making them a good candidate for controlling nausea and vomiting [5].

Special Considerations [5][9]:

- over 60 years of age, you may be more likely to experience side effects from Benadryl and may require a lower dose of Benadryl.
- Benadryl is in the FDA pregnancy category B, but it is contraindicated in nursing mothers.
- pediatric in particular may produce excitation.
- has an atropine-like action
- Because patients can sometimes experience pain at the injection site, rapid heart beat, and shortness of breath when injected, it may be best to dilute Benadryl in 10ml of normal saline and injected slowly over 1-2 minutes.
- Patients may experience feeling of restlessness and a compelling need to move. This is often mistaken for anxiety and is not in any way life threatening.
- Should not be given to patients that have the following:
    - glaucoma
    - a stomach ulcer
    - Dementia
    - Parkinson's

- an enlarged prostate or difficulty urinating
- hyperthyroidism
- hypertension
- heart problems
- or asthma.

Benadryl (diphenhydramine) [8][29]

	Onset	Peak	Duration
Adult >12 yrs IV	Rapid	unknown	4-8hr
	DOSE 10 to 50 mg q2-3hr or 25mg/min Max = 400mg/day		
Geriatric IV	May require dose adjustment		
Pediatric (6-12) IV	**DOSE** 1.25mg/kg Max 150mg/day		

Potential Adverse Effects [8][29]

Sedation/sleepiness	Dizziness	Epigastric distress
Thickening of bronchial secretions	Excitation especially in pediatrics	Hypotension in elderly
Extrapyramidal reaction		

Summary

The use of multimodal approaches in areas like Interventional Radiology and endoscopy suites are rarely used. Perhaps its because the use of opioid analgesics and benzodiazepines have been considered the standard approach to preventing pain and sedation. Other possibilities to consider is multimodal methods just aren't taught in moderate sedation curriculums. But think how beneficial preemptive analgesia and antihistamines can be if utilized. Patients may experience less unwanted side effects, over sedation, lengthen recoveries, and pain during and after the procedure.

Sedative Hypnotics & Dissociative Agents

One of the most frustrating issues with moderate sedation is that not all state boards of nursing across the U.S are consistent with the administration of medications by nurses. This is especially the case with medications such as sedative hypnotics and dissociative agents. Most states in the U.S commonly express the same position on sedative hypnotics and dissociative agents:

> *Drugs such as propofol, ketamine, etomidate, methohexital, and thiopental for the use of sedation and anesthesia, by a registered nurse, present specific safety concerns and may not be appropriate unless trained and completed a Certified Registered Nurse Anesthetist (CRNA) program.*

Other States will allow nurses to manage, titrate, and give under special circumstances such as rapid intubation or palliative care (see box 23). For these reasons I've included the some but not all sedative hypnotic and dissociative agents in this book.

Box 23 — **WV Board of Examiners for Registered Professional Nurses**
Chp. 30, Article 7, Section 15
Oct 22, 2010

It is not within the scope of practice for a professional registered nurse to administer anesthetics such as ketamine, propofol, etomidate, sodium thiopental, methohexial, nitrous oxide, and paralytics, except under the following circumstances:

Managing a continuous infusion of an anesthetic agent or paralytic for a patient who is intubated and ventilated in the acute care setting. Dose titration and bolus of agents to be administered to the intubated and ventilated patient may be implemented by RN's, based upon specific orders or protocols signed by qualified licensed physicians.

- Rapid Sequence Intubation- agents may be administered in the presence of a physician or advanced practiced registered nurse credentialed in emergency airway management and cardio vascular support.

Chapter 30, article 7, section 15 for further explanation

Hypnotics & Other Sedatives

Hypnotics are medications such as barbiturates or anti-anxiety agents, that depresses the activity of the central nervous system. They are used to relieve anxiety and induce sleep [33]. Propofol and Precedex are probably the two most common hypnotics and sedatives used in moderate and deep sedation.

Propofol

Propofol was originally developed by Imperial Chemical Industries as ICI 35868, in the United Kingdom. In 1977, clinical trials of this drug began but ended when anaphylactic reactions occurred. It was reformulated and the reintroduced in 1968, but the U.S FDA did not approve the use of propofol until 2008 [14].

Propofol is classified as a non-barbiturate sedative hypnotic that possesses intrinsic antiemetic effects and lacks analgesic properties. What makes this drug so appealing to sedation providers is its very rapid onset and recovery [9][20]24].

Considerations in the administration of Propofol [9][20][24][37]:

- Not indicated in patients with allergies to eggs, egg products, soybeans or soy products
- Reduce doses in the elderly, hypovolemic and other high risk patients.
- **Capnography should be utilized.** Even at low doses propofol can cause decreased oxygen levels and increased carbon dioxide levels.
- Propofol Infusion Syndrome can occur in adult and pediatric ICU infusions. This syndrome is generally seen when propofol has been administered for prolonged and high-dose infusions (> 5 mg/kg/h for > 24h).
- Some characterizations of this may include:
    - severe metabolic acidosis
    - hyperkalemia
    - Lipemia
    - Rhabdomyolysis
    - Hepatomegaly
    - cardiac and renal failure.
- **Strict aseptic technique must always be used.** Use 70% isopropyl alcohol to disinfect rubber stopper. Propofol has

been associated with microbial contamination and with fever, sepsis, other life-threatening illness, and/or death.

- o **Discard within 6 hrs after spike or immediately when completing a procedure**.
- o As per manufacture, propofol is to be used for sedation of intubated, mechanically ventilated patients in the Intensive Care Unit (ICU), titration of propofol should be performed by persons trained in critical care, cardiopulmonary resuscitation and airway management.

Propofol [20][37]				
	Onset	Peak	Duration	Dose
Adult	30 sec	1 min	2-10 min	Bolus: 10-50mg Titrate: 25-100 mcg/kg/min

Propofol Potential Adverse Reaction [20][37]	
Hypotension	Decreased intracranial pressure and cerebral blood flow.
Respiratory depression/apnea	Pulmonary edema
Airway obstruction	Lactic acidosis due to lipid based
Pain at injection site (reduced by lidocaine)	Green urine
Hiccoughs	Wheezing/coughing

Manufacture Recommendations
as per the manufacture, is used for the purpose of general anesthesia or monitored anesthesia care (MAC) sedation, should be initiated and administered only by persons trained in the specialty of general anesthesia, who is not involved in the conduction of the surgical/diagnostic procedure.

Controversies Regarding Non-anesthesiologist Administered Propofol [24]:

Here is where the topic of administrating propofol gets controversial. Some characteristics of propofol can make it difficult to use for moderate sedation. The problem with propofol is that it is considered unpredictable and therefore been regulated by the FDA as an anesthetic agent. For this reason propofol should be administered by persons trained in the administration of general anesthesia. So unless the a nurse practices in a state that has specifically permits Nurse-administered propofol sedation (NAPS), propofol administered by non-anesthesiologists is considered an off label use, and will do so at their own legal peril.

Non-anesthesiologist administered propofol (NAAP) and Nurse-administered propofol sedation (NAPS).

Even though administration of propofol is not recommended to be given by non-anesthesiologist ,the American College of Gastroenterology, the American Gastroenterological Association and the American Society for Gastrointestinal Endoscopy developed recommendations in 2004, that endorses Non-anesthesiologist administered propofol (NAAP). Non-anesthesiologist administered propofol (NAAP) is the administration of propofol, other than an anesthesia, either by a physician, nurse, or registered nurse under the direction of a physician. The NAAP physician-nurse teams must also possess the training and expertise necessary to rescue patients from severe respiratory complications. Currently there are two models utilized for the administration of propofol by non-anesthesiologists during endoscopic sedation: Nurse-administered Propofol Sedation (NAPS) and Gastroenterologist-directed propofol.

The initial and probably the most utilized model is the Nurse-administered Propofol Sedation (NAPS). This entails the administration of propofol by a registered nurse under the supervision and direction of an endoscopist. The nurse's only responsibilities during the procedure include patient monitoring, administration and titration of propofol ordered by the physician. With NAPS, propofol is the only medication used for moderate sedation.

The second type of nurse-physician model is the Gastroenterologist-directed propofol. With this model The physician and nurse share dosing responsibility. Propofol is combined with other medications such as a benzodiazepine and an opioid to achieve sedation.

Summary

Propofol can be a great medication for sedating patients with endoscopic procedures. However because propofol has characteristics that can not always be controlled, it is not recommended by the manufacture to be given by anyone other than a trained person in the specialty of general anesthesia. Nonetheless, Propofol administered by a non-anesthesiologist such as the NAAP & NAP is considered an off label use and should follow the recommendations endorsed by the American College of Gastroenterology, the American Gastroenterological Association and the American Society for Gastrointestinal Endoscopy. Perhaps in the future we will see a consistent and rigorous training model nation wide that will be debunk any controversy of non-anesthesiologist administered propofol.

Precedex (Dexmedetomidine Hydrochloride)

Precedex was approved by the FDA in 1994 for short term sedation of intubated patients in the intensive or critical care units. Any use under procedural sedation up until 2008, was considered an off label use [10]. After 2008 precedex was welcomed to the procedural sedation world with opens arms. Today it is often seen utilized for procedural sedation in adults and children[27].

What makes this drug so appealing is it's trifecta action of being a hypnotic, sedative, and analgesic. Not only does precedex seem like a one size fits all medication for sedation and analgesic, it also doesn't appear to have any profound adverse effects on respiratory system [37].

Another perk to precedex , by the manufactures (Hospira) recommendations, is that it can be administered to a non-intubated patient for procedural sedation by persons skilled in the management of patients in the intensive care or operating room setting [10]. Although this sounds like good information it also seems pretty grey for non-anesthesiologist sedation teams. Basically it appears that as long as a healthcare professional has ICU, airway management, and cardiopulmonary resuscitation experience then they are allowed to administer precedex to non-intubated patients for sedation at their own risk. Keep in mind that although Hospira makes these recommendations it is ultimately regulated by state and institutions who can administer precedex for procedural sedation.

Considerations for Precedex administration [8][37]:

- Do not exceed infusion over 24 hrs. Tolerance, tachyphylaxis, ARDS, respiratory failure, and agitation can occur.
- Should be administered with caution in patients with advanced heart block and/or severe ventricular dysfunction.
- Antisedan (atipamezole) is a antagonist that rapidly and effectively reverses precedex.
- Rapid IV infusion or bolus can cause clinically significant bradycardia and sinus arrest.
- A decrease in blood pressure and heart rate should be anticipated.
- Precedex has the potential to induce vagal response, anticholinergic agents, like atropine, should be at hand.
- Rate reduction should be consider in the elderly and for those patients with impaired hepatic and renal functions. Precedex has a higher incidence of producing bradycardia and hypotension in these populations.
- Precedex is a Category C and is not recommended for pregnant or lactating women unless potential benefits justify potential risks.
- Precedex should not be used in patients below the age of 18. There have been no clinical studies conducted to determine the safety of administration in the pediatric population.
- Should be administered using a controlled infusion device.

Precedex for Non-intubated Patients Requiring Sedation [31]			
	Onset	Peak	Half-Life
Adult	10-15 min	20-30 min	6 min
Dose	0.5-1mcg/kg/hr loading dose over 10 min. Followed by 0.6mcg/kg/hr with titrations of 0.2-1 mcg/kg/hr		

Precedex Potential Adverse Reactions [8][37]	
Cardiac Arrhythmias Bradycardia & Sinus arrest reported in both the young and healthy adult.	**Tachycardia**
Hypotension more pronounced in geriatric, hypovolemic, chronic hypertensive and diabetic patients	**Nausea / Vomiting**
Hypertension	**Minimal respiratory depression**
Fever	**Hypoxia**

Dissociative Agent

Ketamine is a phencyclidine (PCP) derivative which was first created in 1962 by Dr Calvin Stevens, while researching an alternative to phencyclidine aka PCP or angel dust. During the late 1960's and early 1970's, federal government approved ketamine for human use. At that time it became commonly used as a battlefield anesthetic, especially on battlefields of the Vietnam War. Ketamine became popular for its strong analgesic effect without compromising the patients respiratory status [7][17].

During the late 1970's to mid 1980's ketamine was being used as an illicit drug by new age spiritualists and clubbers. A dose of 1-2mg/kg produced a feeling of floating, hallucinations, and dissociation lasting for about an hour. Larger doses produced a condition known as K-hole, which was the verge of being fully sedated and the feeling of an "out of body experience". Like anything else Ketamine has it's bad sides. It was easily used a s a date rape drug because it often left individuals helpless and confused. It is thought that because of ketamine's recreational use the federal government classified ketamine as a Schedule III controlled substance in August 1999, making it for medical use only [7][17].

Ketamine is another medication that registered nurses should not administer as per many U.S state board of nursing, except under the certain circumstances (see your states requirements). Even though this medication may not be permitted to be administrated by nurses, they may still be asked to recover patients who have received Ketamine. For these reason, it is imperative that registered nurses working in procedural sedation areas be educated on ketamine administration and it's potential adverse reactions.

Ketamine is a rapid acting general anesthetic generally used for deep sedation, but can also be used for other reasons such as palliative care. It is most commonly used for the sedation of pediatric patients because of it's ability to produce profound analgesia and a dissociative state, without compromising the respiratory system.

Considerations for Ketamine administration [9][20][21][33][37]:

- Should be used with caution in patients with hypertension, coronary artery disease and CHF. Ketamine stimulates sympathetic nervous system, exciting the cardiac system, increasing myocardial oxygen consumption.

- Should be used with caution in critically ill patients, they may experience hypotension and a decrease in cardiac output.

- Should not be given to patients with intracranial pressure, open eye surgery, or psychiatric illness. Ketamine induces cerebral vasodilation.

- Ketamine produces an increase in secretions, suction should be readily available. Nausea and vomiting may also occur especially in repeated IM doses.

- Unpleasant **EMERGENCE PHENOMENA** may occur: This phenomena may produce fear, anxiety, combativeness, and excitement, and therefore it should not be given to patients that have been a victim of a traumatic experiences (war, rape, PTSD, etc). This adverse reaction typically occurs in ages 15-65 if given IM. The administration of midazolam (versed) can reduce symptoms. Also provide a quiet and calm environment for recovery.

- **Ketamine is not pharmacologically reversible.**

Ketamine [8][20][37]				
Route	Onset	Peak	Duration	Adult Dose
IV	5 secs	15-30 sec	5-10 min	0.25-1 mg/kg Infusion rate max: 50mcg/kg/min
IM	3-8 min	5-20 min	12-25 min	1-2.5 mg/kg
Half Life for IV dose = 2-3hrs				

Ketamine Potential Adverse Reactions [8][20][37]	
Transient erythema	Bradycardia tachycardia arrhythmias
Anxiety, dysphoria, disorientation, insomnia, flashbacks, hallucinations, and	Nausea and Vomiting Increased salivary secretions
EMERGENCE PHENOMENA Environment must be quiet and calm. Occurs less frequent if given IM	Dependence
Respiratory depression	

Antiemetic Therapy

Nausea and vomiting appears to be a common symptom when performing procedures and administrating opioids to patients . The most common causes maybe from the administration of opioids, increased vagal tone, procedural interventions such as y-90's, pain, decrease cerebral blood flow, and many other etiologic diversities. However, regardless of the etiology of nausea and vomiting, it is imperative to think about an antiemetic therapy for those with increased risk of experiencing these responses. A good physician-nurse team should be able to identify and developed a prophylactic plan based on the patients history, medications, and procedure being performed [9][21].

There are various antiemetic medications and non-pharmaceutical interventions that can potentially diminish a nausea and vomiting experience. Some non-pharmaceutical interventions are the encouragement of a positive environment that avoids anxious smells, sights, movement, and conversations. Other treatments may include providing hydration, providing adequate pain relief, and placement of a nasogastric/oralgastric tube [9][21].

Pharmaceutical antiemetic therapies can reduce gastrointestinal (GI) symptoms and may be administer pre, intra, and post procedure. Some common medications include but are not limited to:

- Compazine
- Phenergan
- and Zofran.

For the following antiemetic medications, only a quick reference will be provided. For more information on these medications please visit http://www.drugs.com/ or any other accurate drug reference.

Compazine (Prochlorperazine)

Considerations in the administration of Compazine [8]:

- Do not administer as bolus
- Inject IV Compazine slowly
- Can be administered undiluted or diluted in isotonic solution
- Do not mix injection with other drugs in syringe
- If injection is spilled on skin, rinse area right away with water to prevent contact dermatitis.

Compazine (Prochlorperazine) [8][9][29]				
Onset	Peak	Duration	Dose	Instructions
10 to 20 min (IM).	4-7 days for antipsychotic effects	3 to 4 h (IM).	5-10mg IV or IM 5mg/min IV Max dose: 10mg IV	Give 5mg first and titrate to effect to no more than max dose.
Adverse reaction: Drowsiness, dizziness, Hyperglycemia; hypoglycemia, Orthostatic hypotension				

Phenergan (Promethazine)

Considerations for Phenergan administration [9][29]:

- Phenergan Injection should not be used in pediatric patients < 2 years of age due of the possibility of a fatal respiratory depression.

- Irritation and severe tissue Injury, Including Gangrene, can occur regardless of route. Patient may experience burning, pain, thrombonphlebitis, and tissue necrosis.

- Best given IM vs. IV

Phenergan (Promethazine) [9][29]				
Onset	Peak	Duration	Dose	Instructions
20 min	4-6 hr	12 or less	12.5-25mg IV or 25-50mg IM	IV inject 25mg/min
Adverse reaction: drowsiness, dry mouth, tinnitus, blurred vision, hypotension, hypertension, nasal stuffiness, lower seizure threshold, gangrene, Neuroleptic Malignant Syndrome				

Zofran (Ondansetron Hydrochloride)

Considerations for administration [8][9][28]:

- For preventive treatment of nausea and vomiting intra and post procedure, it is best to give a dosage of 16 mg (give as two 8-mg Zofran tablets or 16 mg/20ml of Ondansetron), one hour before the procedure.
- Least sedative than Compazine or Phenergan.

Zofran (Ondansetron Hydrochloride) [8][9][39]				
Onset	Peak	Duration	Dose	Instructions
20 min	3.5 hr	8 hr or less	4mg IV	Inject 4mg over 2-5min
Adverse reaction: minimal side effects compared to Phenergan and Compazine.				

Summary

The nausea and vomiting center is located in the medulla of the brain. It is primarily triggered by nervous impulses from, stimulation of higher brain centre, by chemoreceptor triggers zone impulses and by the stomach, intestinal tract, and other portions of the body, resulting in a reflexive activation. There are some patients that may respond to pain, anxiety, medications, and complex procedures, in a way that elicits the nausea and vomiting response. For preventative antiemetic therapy, it is beneficial during the pre-procedure phase that the patient is assessed for any current nausea and past history of emetic responses from opioids or procedures.

Reference:

1. *Acetaminophen (iv)*. (n.d.). Retrieved from http://www.drugguide.com
2. Ativan http://www.drugs.com/pro/ativan.htm
3. *As morphine turns 200, drug that blocks*. (2005, May 19). Retrieved from http://opioids.com/morphine/200-anniv.html
4. Baskett, T., & Hamilton, G. (2000). In the arms of morpheus the development of. *Anaesth, 47*(4), 367-74.

5. Becker, D. E. (2012). Pharmacodynamic considerations for moderate and deep sedation. *Anesth Prog*, *59*(1), 28-42. Retrieved from http://www.ncbi.nlm.nih.gov

6. Chen, J., Ko, T., Wen, Y., Wu , S., Chou, Y., Yien, H., & Kuo, C. (2009). Opioid-sparing effects of ketorolac and its correlation with the recovery of postoperative bowel function in colorectal surgery patients: a prospective randomized double-blinded study. *Clin J Pain*, *25*(6), 485-9.

7. *Center for substance abuse research*. (n.d.). Retrieved from http://www.cesar.umd.edu/cesar/drugs/ketamine.asp

8. Drugs.com (n.d). Retrieved from http://www.drugs.com/

9. ESLINGER, M. R. (n.d.). Moderate sedation certification. Retrieved from www.sedationcertification.com

10. *Fda approves new indication for precedex*. (n.d.). Retrieved from http://www.drugs.com/newdrugs/fda-approves-new-indication-hospira-s-precedex-dexmedetomidine-hcl-1166.html

11. Felden, L.; C. Walter; S. Harder; R.-D. Treede; H. Kayser; D. Drover; G. Geisslinger; J. Lötsch (22). "Comparative Clinical Effects of Hydromorphone and Morphine". *British Journal of Anesthesia* 107 (3): 319–328

12. Fentanyl history. (2013, July 23). *News Medical*. Retrieved from Fentanyl historyhttp://www.news-medical.net/health/Fentanyl-History.aspx

13. History of morphine. (2013, August 13). *News Medical*. Retrieved from http://www.news-medical.net/health/Morphine-History.aspx

14. *the history of surgery and anesthesia* . (n.d.). Retrieved from http://www.historyofsurgery.co.uk/Web Pages/0185.htm

15. Kaiko, R., Foley, K., Grabinski, P., Heidrich, G., Rogers, A., Inturrisi, C., & Reidenberg, M. (1983). Central nervous system excitatory effects of meperidine in cancer patients. *Annals of Neurology* , *13*(2), 180-185.

16. Kanto JH. (May 1982). "Use of benzodiazepines during pregnancy, labour and lactation, with particular reference to pharmacokinetic considerations". *Drugs.* 23 (5): 354–80

17. *Ketamine: the story.* (n.d.). Retrieved from http://www.thesite.org/drinkanddrugs/drugculture/wheredrugscomefrom/ketamine]

18. *Ketorolac.* (n.d.). Retrieved from http://www.drugs.com/mtm/ketorolac.html

19. *Ketorolac and tromethamine.* (n.d.). Retrieved from http://medical-dictionary.thefreedictionary.com/ketorolac tromethamine

20. Kost, M. (2004). Moderate sedation/analgesia. (2nd ed.). St. Louis: Saunders.

21. Lazear, S. E. (2011). Moderate sedation/analgesia. Sacremento, California: CME Resource. Retrieved from http://www.netce.com/courseoverview.php?courseid=751

22. Lewis, A. N. (2012, January). Iv acetaminophen (ofirmev). *Pharmacy Times*, DOI: www.pharmacytimes.com

23. Michaelis, M; Schölkens, B; Rudolphi, K; Bermward S, Rudolphi K (April 2007). "An anthology from Naunyn-Schmiedeberg's archives of pharmacology". *Naunyn-Schmiedeberg's Archives of Pharmacology* (Springer Berlin) 375 (2): 81–84

24. *Non-anesthesiologist administered propofol (naap).* (n.d.). Retrieved from http://www.sgna.org/Issues/SedationFactsorg/SedationAdministration/Agents_DeliveryMethods/Naap.aspx

25. Norman, P. H., Daley, M. D., & Linsedy, R. W. (2001). Preemptive analgesic effects of ketorolac in ankle fracture surgery. *Anesthesiology, 94*(4), 599-603.

26. Ong, K., Seymour, R., Chen, F., & Ho, V. (2004). Preoperative ketorolac has a preemptive effect for postoperative third molar surgical pain. *Int J Oral Maxillofac Surg , 33*(8), 771-6.

27. Orlewicz, M. (2013, May 28). Procedural sedation. *Medscape*, Retrieved from http://emedicine.medscape.com/article/109695-overview

28. Pasero, C., & Stannard, D. (2013). The role of intravenous acetaminophen in acute pain management. *Pain management Nursing , 13*(2), 107-124.

29. *Physician desk reference*. (n.d.). Retrieved from http://www.pdr.net

30. Porucznik, M. A. (2010, July). Two views on multimodal pain management. *AAOS Now*, Retrieved from http://www.aaos.org/news/aaosnow/jul10/clinical8.asp

31. *Precedx dosing guide* . (n.d.). Retrieved from http://www.precedex.com/wp-content/uploads/2010/02/Dosing_Guide.pdf]

32. *SedationFacts.org.* Sleep Apnea and other Sedation Complications. September 29,2008. http://sedation.sgna.org

33. *Sedative hypnotic*. (n.d.). Retrieved from http://www.thefreedictionary.com/sedative-hypnotic

34. *Short history of valium*. (2013). Retrieved from http://www.buydiazepam.net/history.html

35. Sullivan, P. (2005, October 1). Inventor of valium, once the most often prescribed drug, dies. *Washington Post*. Retrieved from http://www.washingtonpost.com/wp-dyn/content/article/2005/09/30/AR2005093001963.html

36. *Toradol*. (n.d.). Retrieved from http://www.fundinguniverse.com/company-histories/roche-bioscience-history/]

37. Urman, R. D, & Kaye, A. D. (2012). Moderate and deep sedation in clinical practice. New York: Cambridge University Press.

Other resources:

38. Hevesi, D. (2007, September 27). *The New York Times*. Retrieved from http://www.nytimes.com/2007/09/29/business/29rieveschl.html?ref=health&_r=0

Chapter 8

Special Populations

ASA >3
Age Specific (Pediatric & Geriatric)
Obese
Pregnancy/lactating
Sleep Apnea
COPD
Chronic Opioid use/ Methadone
Drug & ETOH abuse

Not every patient that a nurse is going to administer moderate sedation to and monitor is going to be the picture of perfect health (ASA I). There will be times when high risk patients will be sedated. Either because the patient had a poor pre-evaluation, did not have an anesthesia consult ordered as recommended, or the patient is simply teetering on the GREY line of being a candidate for moderate sedation. These types of cases leave nursing in a sticky position and with legal ramifications if not addressed appropriately.

High risk patients can define as the following [1][2]:
- High risk for procedural complication
- High risk for sedation complication
- High risk for sedation failure

The most common reasons for sedation failure are from [1] [2]:
- Drug overdose
- Polypharmacy
- Poor Patient Selection
- Inadequate Monitoring
- Under Appreciation of Potential Drug Interactions
- Inadequate Preoperative Assessment, especially for ill patients in hospital Setting

The best nursing defenses for high risk patients are:
- Education
- Training
- and a thorough pre-evaluation assessment.

ASA >3

In 1963 the American Society of Anesthesiologists (ASA) adopted a five category physical status classification system to help determine a patients overall physical health or sickness preoperatively. Today it is highly regarded by regulatory bodies, hospitals, accrediting boards and other healthcare groups as a scale to predict risk for complications during surgery [4]. Because this scale predicts the possibility of adverse effects it has been recommended for the use in determining candidates for moderate sedation. Patients that fall in the classes 1-2 are considered good candidates for moderate sedation. Those patients that are considered classes 3 and above however carry a higher risk and may need consultation from anesthesia services to better determine if moderate sedation is appropriate [3]. A patient with an ASA classification of 3 and above is described as the following:

ASA 3
- A patient with severe systemic disease, not incapacitating
- Poorly controlled hypertension. Diabetes, ESRD, past MI, CVA, Cardiac stents, dialysis, EJ of 40%, multiple medications for cardiac, respiratory and/or metabolic disorders. Metastatic disease with some interference with function. Pneumonia

This may be divided into STABLE and UNSTABLE categories:
Stable:
- Controlled insulin-dependent diabetic with hypertension and mild renal disease. A child with congenital heart disease stable on digoxin and lasix.

Unstable:
- Frequent asthma attacks needing ER visits or intubation. Brittle, or difficult to control, insulin dependent diabetic. Severe COPD, on multiple inhalers and difficulty breathing in supine position

ASA 4

- A patient with severe systemic disease that is a constant threat to life. e.g.
- Metastatic disease with severe organ dysfunction. Severe hypertension with angina.
- Recent history of MI, TIA, cardiac stents: continuing symptoms of ischemic or severe valve dysfunction. Implanted ICD, EF of 25%, sepsis, organ insufficiency

ASA 5

- A moribund patient who is not expected to survive.
- Poorly responsive cardiogenic shock
- Ruptured abdominal or thoracic aneurism, intracranial bleed, and ischemic bowel.

Every nurse that provides moderate sedation should be familiar with the ASA physical status classification scale and have the ability to apply this tool when assessing their patients. The also the nurse providing moderate sedation should posses the skill to determine if their patient is at high risk for complications and/or above the nurses scope of practice.

Reference:

1. The Durham VAMC Patient Safety Center of Inquiry (PSCI). (2011, march 29). Moderate sedation toolkit for non-anesthesiologists. Retrieved from http://www.patientsafety.gov/pubs.html
2. ESLINGER, M. R. (n.d.). Moderate sedation certification. Retrieved from www.sedationcertification.com
3. Lazear, S. E. (2011). Moderate sedation/analgesia. Sacremento, California: CME Resource. Retrieved from http://www.netce.com/courseoverview.php?courseid=751
4. Owens, W. D. (2001). American society of anesthesiologist's physical status classification system is not a risk classification system. *Anesthesiology, 94*(2), 378.

Age Specific (Pediatric & Geriatric)
Pediatric

This book is written for those nurses sedating adult patients, but the question in hand is what patients are considered an adult or pediatric patient? Not every institution and organization interprets a pediatric patient the same way. The American Academy of Pediatrics defines a pediatric patient as a newborn to age 21 see box 15[2]. The American Heart Association considers a child over the age of 8 and older adults for Cardio-Pulmonary Resuscitation (CPR)[1]. The U.S Department of Health and Human Services considers adolescences 11-18yrs of age, and adults are 18 yrs and older[9]. Other literature suggests that most adolescence are generally developmentally and intellectually similar to an adult [10]. So as you can see there isn't a real cut and dry answer to this question .

Box 15	Pediatric Population in Sub-groups (Per AAP)[2]
Newborn	Less than 1 day old
Neonate	Less than 30 days old
Infants	1-12 months
Children	1-12 yrs old
Adolescent	13-19 yrs old
Young Adult	20-21 yrs old

http://sedationcertification.com/resources/sedation-medications/pediatric sedation/

Suggestions

When deciding what patient fits into the adult population vs. pediatric, keep in a mind that the ASA states intravenous sedation may be administered to pediatric patients greater than 9 months of age who are evaluated as a Class I or Class II [3]. Also think about what makes the pediatric population so challenging. There are many anatomic, physiologic and psychological differences among pediatric patients 2yrs old and older [2].

Here are other suggestions to this ambiguous area which may answer questions pertaining to sedation of pediatric/adult patients:

- o It can be left black & white. Perform moderate sedation on adults based on the AAP (17-21 yrs old), government

definition (18rs old and older), or the institutions policy[2][9].
- Sedation of adolescence can be performed ONLY IF:
    - Both the nurse and physician are privileged to do so by their healthcare institution and state.
    - both the nurse and privilege physician agree.
    - both the nurse and privileged physician have advance training in pediatric care and have been trained in age appropriate cardio-pulmonary rescue, such as PALS [10].
    - Moderate sedation is titrated per weight [4].
    - The adolescent is an ASA of I and II only [4]

Guidelines

In the effort of establishing consistency and safety for the administration of moderate sedation to pediatric patients, the American Academy of Pediatrics, American Society of Anesthesiologist, American Academy of Pediatric Dentists and the Joint Commission Accreditation of Healthcare Organizations issued a set of guidelines for pediatric sedation (box 16)[8].

Box 16	*Guidelines for Sedation in Children* [5][8]
•	No administration of sedation without medical supervision
•	Pre-sedation evaluation for underlying medical or surgical conditions that could increase risk from sedation.
•	Appropriate pre-procedure fasting for elective procedures (ASA NPO Guidelines).
•	Airway examination to identify abnormalities that could increase the potential for airway obstruction.
•	Thorough understanding of pharmacokinetics and pharmacodynamic effects of sedation medication.
•	Appropriate monitoring during and after procedure.

• Properly equipped and staff recovery area.
• Recovery to point of consciousness before discharge and appropriate discharge instructions.

http://www.sgna.org/issues/sedationfactsorg/specialcircumstances/pediatrics.aspx

Candidates

Patients who are in ASA classes I and II are frequently considered appropriate candidates for minimal, moderate, or deep sedation. Children in ASA classes III and IV, special needs children, and those with anatomic airway abnormalities, present concerns that require additional consideration, mainly for moderate and deep sedation. Practitioners are encouraged to consult with appropriate subspecialists and/or an anesthesiologist for patients at increased risk of experiencing adverse sedation events because of their underlying medical/surgical conditions.

Considerations in the Pediatric Population[5][8]

Many medications utilized for pediatric sedation have not been fully evaluated and approved by the FDA, and are often given "off label". Therefore, the clinician must recognize limitations and seek to define safe sedation appropriately.

- Awareness of age-appropriate vital signs is vital for all ages, see box 17 [7]
- Children 1-5 yr of age are at most risk, even though they have no severe underlying disease. Respiratory depression and obstruction are the most frequent causes of adverse events. Pediatric patients also have a faster oxygen desaturation time than adults. Oxygen de-saturation is known to be the most frequently reported complication.
- **Children are not to be mistaken as little people**. They have physiological differences in anatomy compared to adults. Such differences include: larger tongues, narrow oral-pharyngeal passages, less alveolar space, increased metabolic rate (resulting in higher oxygen consumption), hepatic and renal function are less developed, thinner skin, increased tendency to become hypoglycemic when fasting, and neurologically not fully developed under age 10 yrs [8]

- 100 % O2 should be administered when heart rate decreases [8].
- Pediatric patients should be kept warm to prevent hypothermia.
- Sedation should be administered based on patient weight and titrated by response to sedation.
- Children have Increased renal/hepatic blood flow-faster drug clearance. Higher doses of medication may be needed in the preschool, elementary school aged and pre-teen children.

In summary, providing moderate sedation to a pediatric patient is not so much age dependent as it is state regulated and training dependent. If a nurse has worked in the Neonatal Intensive Care Unit then he or she will probably be comfortable with sedating a pediatric patient. However, if a nurse has only been employed in working with the adult population then he or she may find that they are only competent to administer moderate sedation to those above the age of 13 or even 18 yrs of age.

Box 17   **Pediatric Vital Sign Chart**

Age	Resp rate	Heart rate	Systolic (B/P)	Diastolic (B/P)
Neonate	40	140	65	45
12 months	30	120	95	65
3 yrs	25	100	100	70
12 yrs	20	80	110	60

(Source: Morgan, GE, Jr. and Mikhail, MS. (1996). Clinical anesthesiology. Stamford, Connecticut. Appleton and Lange, p. 727).

References:
1. *Adult-fun cpr training.* (n.d.). Retrieved from http://www.funcpr.com/adultchildinfantcprchart.htm
2. American Academy of Pediatrics. Guidelines for pediatric perioperative anesthesia environment (re9820). *Pediatrics.* 1999;103:512-515
3. Cote, C. J. M. (2006). Guidelines for monitoring and management of pediatric patients during and after sedation for therapeutic and diagnostic procedures: An update.

American academy of pediatrics, American academy of pediatric dentists. *Pediatrics, 118*(6), 2587-2602.

4. *Definition of an older or elderly person.* (2013). Retrieved from http://www.who.int/healthinfo/survey/ageingdefnolder/en/index.html

5. The Durham VAMC Patient Safety Center of Inquiry (PSCI). (2011, march 29). Moderate sedation toolkit for non-anesthesiologists. Retrieved from http://www.patientsafety.gov/pubs.html

6. ESLINGER, M. R. (n.d.). Moderate sedation certification. Retrieved from www.sedationcertification.com

7. Guidelines for Monitoring and Management of Pediatric Patients During and After Sedation for Therapeutic and Diagnostic Procedures: An Update. American Academy of Pediatrics, American Academy of Pediatric Dentists, Cote, C.J, MD, Wilson, S/ DMD, MA, PhD the Workgroup on Sedation. Pediatrics Vol 118 No.6 December 2006 pp 2587-260

8. Kost, M. (2004). Moderate sedation/analgesia. (2nd ed.). St. Louis: Saunders.

9. *Pediatric Sedation.* (2013). Retrieved from http://sedationcertification.com/resources/sedation-medications/pediatric-sedation/

10. http://sedationcertification.com/resources/sedation-medications/pediatric-sedation/

11. http://sedation.sgna.org

12. United States Department of Health & Human Services. (n.d.). *What is adolescence.* Retrieved from http://www.hhs.gov/opa/familylife/tech_assistance/etraining/adolescent_brain/Overview/what_is_adolescence/index.html

13. Urman, Richard D. and Kaye, Alan D. Moderate and Deep Sedation in Clinical Practice. Cambridge University Press, 2012.

Geriatric

According to the World Health Organization (WHO) the accepted age to define the elderly or geriatric is sixty five and older. Although this age varies from country to country this seems to be the accepted age in western civilization. The determination generally developed from the age in which individuals retire and receive pensions from their careers [1][8]. Regardless of the exact age of the older patient, what needs to be taken into consideration is that as a person ages their physiologic and psychological condition changes.

Physiologic changes elderly patients experience [2][3][6][8]:
- Decreased blood volume
- Decreased vascular compliance and heart rate
- Upper airway protective reflexes diminish. Decreased ability to cough and ability to respond to hypoxia and hypercarbia.
- Loss of chest wall elasticity and muscle strength, Increased chest wall rigidity and residual volume.
- Decreased glomerular filtration rate (GFR) prolongs the amount of time drugs are cleared by the kidneys.
- Most have co morbidities such as CAD, HTN, COPD, DM, cognitive impairment, and renal insufficiency.
- Most are also on many medications due to their co-morbidities.

Considerations that need to be taken when administering moderate sedation to geriatric patients include but are not limited to the following [2][3][5][6][8]:
- Positioning
  - The physiological changes of the skin and the blood thinning agents that the elderly population receive, puts this population at risk for skin tears and bruises. Thinning of the skin and the loss of fat can also make bony prominences or arthritic areas painful if not cushioned appropriately.
- Medications
  - Because most geriatric patients are hypovolemic and have reduced renal & hepatic functions, reaction to medications may be delayed include a delay in fat

soluble drugs and hypersensitivity in water soluble drugs like, CNS depressants. Because of these changes, the most likely problem to encounter in this population is over-sedation. Having knowledge of this, the nurse should ensure that lower doses of moderate sedation be administered, at a slow rate, and an overall low accumulation.

- Common reactions to medications may include:
  - Hypotension
    - It is believed that this population is chronically volume depleted due to diuretic therapy.
  - Confusion and delirium
  - Respiratory depression
    - the elderly patient is profoundly at risk for hypoxemia due to decreased respiratory drive that occurs with normal ageing.
  - Increased risk of aspiration due to decreased gag reflex
  - Dsyrhythmia
    - Is a common occurrence during sedation and can be often corrected with oxygen administration.
- Anatomical Changes
  - The use of dentures may greatly affect the ability to perform ventilation. An Ambu bag and ventilation mask may not seal well if dentures are removed prior to procedure. Arthritis of the neck can also play a factor in the way airway rescue takes place. A stiff or painful neck may cause difficulty in performing head-tilt chin lift.

The geriatric population is more frequently seen by nurses for diagnostic and interventional procedures. This group is by far the riskiest group to sedate. Geriatric patients come with a wide range of medications and co-morbities that a typical adult patient would not have. The nurse needs to keep in mind to slowly titrate the moderate sedation medication and be particularly vigilant about their monitoring with this group. Lastly, although the main responsibility for the pre-assessment is to be conducted by the physician, it never hurts for the nurse to perform his or her own quick assessment to ensure that moderate sedation is in fact the best method of sedation.

Reference:
1. *Definition of an older or elderly person.* (2013). Retrieved from http://www.who.int/healthinfo/survey/ageingdefnolder/en/index.html
2. The Durham VAMC Patient Safety Center of Inquiry (PSCI). (2011, march 29). Moderate sedation toolkit for non-anesthesiologists. Retrieved from http://www.patientsafety.gov/pubs.html
3. ESLINGER, M. R. (n.d.). Moderate sedation certification. Retrieved from www.sedationcertification.com
4. Kost, M. (2004). Moderate sedation/analgesia. (2nd ed.). St. Louis: Saunders.
5. Lazear, S. E. (2011). Moderate sedation/analgesia. Sacramento, California: CME Resource. Retrieved from http://www.netce.com/courseoverview.php?courseid=751
6. http://sedation.sgna.org
7. United States Department of Health & Human Services. (n.d.). *What is adolescence*. Retrieved from http://www.hhs.gov/opa/familylife/tech_assistance/etraining/adolescent_brain/Overview/what_is_adolescence/index.html
8. Urman, Richard D. and Kaye, Alan D. Moderate and Deep Sedation in Clinical Practice. Cambridge University Press, 2012.

Pregnancy and Lactation

There seems to be few studies, education, and practice guidelines on the sedation of pregnant patients. For these reasons it is not without certainty, known whether the administration of moderate sedation during pregnancy places mother and fetus at risk for complications. There also is the fact that pregnancy itself changes the anatomy and physiology of women, making her a high risk for compromised airway. These circumstances surrounding pregnancy often make it difficult for the moderate sedation nurse to feel comfortable sedating this population.

Anatomic and physiologic changes of a pregnant patient[2][3]:

- Nasal and mucus membranes become engorged leading to narrowing of airway.
- There is a compensatory increase in minute ventilation to meet maternal and fetus oxygen demand
- Reduced lung capacity occurs as diaphragm becomes elevated and as fetus enlarges increasing the risk of maternal hypoxemia
- Heart rate increases to 90-100 beats per minute
- Cardiac output increase up to 40% and is affected by positioning
- Systolic blood pressure can drop and supine hypotension may develop.
- Gastro-intestinal motility and food absorption decreases
- In the 2nd and 3rd trimester the vena cava and aorta become compressed by the uterus increasing the risk for maternal tachycardia and fetal distress.

Risks of procedure and sedation include [2][3]:

- over sedation resulting in hypotension and hypoventilation.
- compression of the vena cava by the uterus can leading to decreased blood flow and fetal hypoxia.
- terratogenesis to the fetus from medications given to the mother and/or ionizing radiation.
- premature birth of fetus
- aspiration

- premature contractions
- dehydration from NPO

Recommendations and Considerations [2][3]:

- Procedures performed during pregnancy should be done only when the indication for the procedure is clear and less invasive diagnostic or therapeutic modalities have been attempted or do not exist. The greatest risks for adverse effects in fetal development occur in the first trimester. If possible, it is best practice to postpone any procedures until after second trimester of pregnancy.
- Informed consent should include risks to the fetus as well as the mother.
- Consultation with obstetrician and/or anesthesia regarding medication use should be considered. High risk pregnancies should be performed by anesthesia services.
- Before the 24 weeks of gestation, it maybe suggested to confirm the presence of the fetal heart rate by doppler before sedation and after the procedure.
- After 24 wks of fetal gestation, it may be suggested to simultaneously monitor fetal heart rate and uterine contraction before and after the procedure.
- Consider fetal monitoring by obstetric nurse, esp. in high risk pregnancies. Decision to monitor fetal heart rate should be individualized and should be dependent on gestational age of fetus and available resources.
- Patient should be positioned in left pelvic tilt or left lateral position to avoid compression of the vena cava and aorta.
- Drug dosing can be the same as a non-pregnant female, however to minimize potential risk of teratogenic effects it is suggested to administer sedatives and analgesic agents in the smallest effective dose as possible.
- The U.S. Food and Drug Administration categorizes drugs into five groups (A,B,C,D, and X) based on the evidence of their safety during pregnancy. Category A is safe to use in pregnant women while category D demonstrates positive evidence of fetal abnormalities and the use of any drug in this category is contraindicated in women who are or may be

pregnant. In general, most common sedatives and analgesics fall within categories B & C. See box 18.

Box 18 Commonly used Medications for Sedation [3]		
Drugs	**FDA Category**	**Comments**
Narcotic Analgesics		
Meperidine	B	Does not appear to be teratogenic in two studies. Preferred over Fentanyl and morphine
Fentanyl	C	Shown to be safe in humans when given in small doses. Rapid onset and faster recovery time than meperidine
Morphine	C	No added risk of congenital malformations in humans has been linked with the use of morphine in pregnancy. There are no controlled data in human pregnancy. Morphine should only be given when benefit outweighs risk.
Benzodiazepines		
Midazolam	D	Avoid giving in 1st trimester. Has not been reported to be linked with congenital abnormalities. Is the chosen benzodiazepine when meperidine is not enough.
Diazepam	D	Should be avoided in pregnant patients. Has been know to cause cleft palate and neurobehavioral disorders

Reversal Agents		
Naloxone	B	Has not shown to be teratogenic. Use only in events of respiratory depression, hypotension or unresponsiveness
Flumazenil	C	Not a teratogenic, but has produced neurobehavioral changes in male rats while in utero

Reference: Safety in Pregnancy of Commonly Used Medications for Endoscopic Sedation, http://sedation.sgna.org

Lactation

Sedating a patient who is breast feeding doesn't seem to be nearly as difficult to address as pregnancy. The primary concern in those patients who are lactating and are receiving IV moderate sedation seems to be the risk of transferring drugs to the infant through the milk. Most nurses and institutions are familiar with the PUMP and DUMP method to help eliminate the potential harms of certain sedatives and analgesics. There are however some additional recommendations to think about in regard to procedural preparation and discharge.

Pre-procedure recommendations

- If the patient's baby is entirely fed from the breast, it is important that the patient be referred to a lactation consultant prior to the procedure and sedation, to ensure that coordination of supplementary feedings and arrangements for a breast pump have been made temporally post procedure [1].
- Arrangements should be made so that nursing the infant can occur immediately prior to the procedure and/or expression and freezing of breast milk can occur.
- The patient should be provided and educated on medication elimination times. A medication list such as the one in box 19 may be appropriate before or at discharge.

Box 19   Lactation Guidelines for Commonly Used Drugs

Drugs	Comments
Meperidine	o Concentrated in breast milk up to 24 hrs after administration o May have neurobehavioral effects on infant
Fentanyl	o Breast feeding may continued after maternal administration. The American academy of pediatrics considers Fentanyl to be compatible with breast feeding. o Excreted in milk up to 10hrs but in very low concentrations o Preferred over Meperidine
Morphine	o Morphine is excreted into human milk in trace amounts. Adverse effects in the nursing infant are unlikely. o Morphine is considered compatible with breast-feeding by the American Academy of Pediatrics. o Meperidine is preferred
Midazolam	o Effects on infant unknown o Takes up to 4hrs to excrete after maternal administration
Propofol	o Excreted in milk with maximum concentration 4-5 hrs post administration o The period of prohibition has not been determined o Effects are unknown to infant
Naloxone and Flumazenil	Effects unknown to infant

Reference:
1. The Durham VAMC Patient Safety Center of Inquiry (PSCI). (2011, march 29). Moderate sedation toolkit for non-anesthesiologists. Retrieved from http://www.patientsafety.gov/pubs.html
2. Griese, M. (2011, August 1). Conscious sedation and breastfeeding: Recommendations for patients. *Medications and Vaccines*, Retrieved from http://kellymom.com/bf/can-i-breastfeed/meds/sedation/
3. Lazear, S. E. (2011). Moderate sedation/analgesia. Sacramento, California: CME Resource. Retrieved from http://www.netce.com/courseoverview.php?courseid=751
4. Pregnant & Lactating Women http://www.sgna.org/issues/sedationfactsorg/specialcircumstances/pregnant.aspx

The Bariatric Patient

According to the Center of Disease Control, from 2009-2010, 35.7% of adults and 16.9% children in America were considered obese. That's 78 million adults and 12.5 million children. According to the data collected, those individuals over the age of sixty held the highest obesity percentage. Any person with a BMI of 40 and above was considered morbidly obese [4] [7]. The obese patient can present a variety of challenges for health care providers and the institutions caring for them. Physician-nurse teams, for example, providing moderate sedation find that the obese patient can be very risky to sedate and manage due to their complex co-morbidities and physiological changes.

Common co-morbidities associated with obesity:

- Heart disease
- Diabetes
- Cancer
- Asthma
- Sleep Apnea or OSA

Physiological changes and suggested considerations [1][3][5][6][7]**:**

Obesity causes several health morbidities that affect the cardiovascular, endocrine, and respiratory systems. The system that is most critically affected in an obese patient is the pulmonary and airway system.

- Extra weight constricts chest wall expansion, increases airway resistance and decreases total lung capacity. This patient population also consumes more oxygen than the average healthy adult, making them more of a risk for faster desaturation than a normal sized adult. The ARIN states that the obese patient's oxygen de-saturation rate can occur three times faster than a patient with a normal weight.

- Capnography may be beneficial in early detection of poor ventilation.

- Oxygen administration from the beginning of the procedure may be a consideration.

- The physical changes of increased tissue around the face, pharyngeal and jaw makes airway management difficult. A small mouth, narrowed airway, thick neck, and large tongue make it difficult to provide proper rescue breathing with a bag mask and more than likely a difficult intubation if needed.

    - Narrowing of the upper airway and loss of upper airway muscles can lead to Obstructive Sleep Apnea (OSA). Approximately 60-90 % of people with a BMI greater than 30kg/m2 have OSA.

        - Anesthesia should be consulted.

        - The STOP-BANG questionnaire (see appendix) is a screening tool for identifying OSA in obese patients who have not yet been diagnosed with OSA. This tool helps determine whether obese patients are at a higher risk for complications to sedation during the procedure.

        - If a patient uses BIPAP at home, it may be beneficial if the patient uses BIPAP during and after a moderately sedated procedure. A BIPAP device keeps the airway of the patient open via pressure, allowing him or her to breathe easily while sleeping **It is important to be aware that a BIPAP is not to be mistaken for a ventilator!**

    - Gastroparesis and increased abdominal pressure is believed to occur in this population. Reflux and the delay of digestion can potentially put this type of patient at risk for aspiration.

    - Reducing the possibility of aspiration can be accomplished by, having the patient follow an 8 hr NPO guideline, recommended by the ASA, and/or administer an intravenous H2 blocker and a GI stimulant, such as Reglan (metoclopramide). Keep in mind the onset of action when preparing the patient for a moderate sedation case. Have them arrive with enough time for the patient to reap the benefits of these medications.

- Onset of action of metoclopramide is 1 to 3 minutes following an intravenous dose, 10 to 15 minutes following intramuscular administration, and 30 to 60 minutes following an oral dose; effects persist for 1-2 hrs [6].

- Onset of H2-blockers is about 1 hr. The half life is generally 2-3 hrs, and can potentially last for 12 hrs [6].

- The obese patient has more adipose tissue than a person that of normal weight. This causes an obese individual to have a longer elimination time for lipophilic drugs such as, Fentanyl.

- The obese patient is also has an increase sensitivity to CNS depressants.

  - Slow titration of moderate sedation medication in very small increments is vital.
  - Decreasing dosing to 30-50% is recommended

- Monitoring difficulties' can also arise from the patients physical changes.

  - Blood pressure cuffs usually don't fit well on the obese patient's upper arm. Using a cuff on the forearm is recommended.

The most likely problems encountered in this population is hypoxia, upper airway obstruction and difficulty in airway rescue. For these reasons the obese patient is a high risk patient to sedate. The importance of a thorough pre-procedure assessment is crucial in the planning of sedation and outcome. Special devices may be needed for the procedure such as BIPAP or CPAP. All members of the sedating team should have special education related to the needs and risks of the patient. If the patients co-morbities dictate a higher level of care for patient safety than anesthesia should be consulted.

Reference:

1. The American Radiologic and Imaging Nursing (ARIN) https://www.arinursing.org/dmdocuments/ARIN_ClinicalGuideline_ModerateSedationandAnalgesia_2009.pdf
2. Bariatric Patient Safety in the Imaging Environment. (2009) Association of Radiologic and Imaging Nursing https://www.arinursing.org/index.php?option=com_content&task=view&id=202&Itemid=267
3. ESLINGER, M. R. (n.d.). Moderate sedation certification. Retrieved from www.sedationcertification.com
4. Ogden, C. L., Carroll,, M. D., Kit,, B. K., & Flega, K. M. (2012). Prevalence of obesity in the united states, 2009–2010. *NCHS Data Brief*, (28), Retrieved from http://www.cdc.gov/nchs/data/databriefs/db82.pdf
5. SGNA, Sedation Facts http://sedation.sgna.org
6. Reglan. drugs.com http://www.drugs.com/pro/reglan.html
7. Urman, Richard D. and Kaye, Alan D. Moderate and Deep Sedation in Clinical Practice. Cambridge University Press, 2012.

Sleep Apnea

Approximately 12-18 million Americans have Obstructive Sleep Apnea (OSA), but roughly 82-90% of people go undiagnosed [4]. OSA primarily affects men between the ages of 30 and 50. It occurs when air passage in the upper respiratory tract becomes obstructed, generally by the pharynx, during sleep. It is often thought that obese or bariatric individuals suffer from this condition, patients do not have to be obese to have sleep apnea. Sleep apnea is more common in people who smoke, drink alcohol and /or live in higher altitudes [1]. If an undiagnosed patient with OSA undergoes moderate sedation they are at a greater risk for airway complications than a non OSA patient.

The key to addressing undiagnosed OSA is through educating the sedation team and by performing a thorough pre-procedure assessment of the patient.

Education of the Sedation Team

Educating those involved in the sedation process on the identification of OSA is a crucial. The healthcare individuals administering moderate sedation should know the risks associated with OSA and the factors indicating the possibility of OSA.

The risks associated with OSA include [2]:

- Increase post-operative complication rate
- Increase need for intensive care intervention
- Prolong hospital stay

Indicating factors and physiologic changes of OSA [2]:

- Redundant adipose and soft tissue narrowing the airway
- Neck circumference greater than 17 inches for men or 16 inches for women
- Tonsillar hypertrophy
- Recurrent snoring
- Observed suspension in breathing during sleep
- Awakens from sleep with a choking sensation
- Somnolence esp. during the day
- BMI greater than 35

Patients with advance disease process may develop obesity hypoventilation syndrome, which can progress to PICKWICKIAN

SYNDROME. This syndrome is characterized by gross obesity, periodic breathing, even when awake, somnolence, hypoxemia, hypercapnea, polycythemia and pulmonary hypertension.

Recommendations to consider when moderately sedating an OSA patient [3][4][5]

- During pre-procedure assessment the nurse and physician should conduct a mallampati assessment and a STOP BANG screening (see appendix).
- OSA patients have an increased sensitivity to CNS depressants. Medications used for sedation should be titrated slowly in response to respiratory ventilation and O2saturation.
- Dexmedetomidine (Precedex) is the most ideal sedative for OSA patients due to its non-respiratory depressant activity.
- If possible patients should be kept in a lateral position while moderately sedating.
- CPAP (Continuous Positive Airway Pressure) and BIPAP may be used during and after procedures to improve patient ventilation and airway patency. CPAP stents the upper airway, decrease apnea frequency and enhances sleep continuity. **CPAP and BIPAP must not be mistaken for a VENTILAOR! The CPAP/BIPAP machine cannot breathe for a patient. Paralytics must not be used.**
- The American Society of Anesthesiologist advises the use of CO2 monitoring during moderate and deep sedation.

Due to the high number of undiagnosed OSA patients, it is imperative to conduct a detailed pre-procedure assessment. Undiagnosed OSA maybe identified by such screening tools as the STOP-BANG tool and physical exam. Both are used to recognize anatomical and physical indicators of OSA (see appendix for STOP BANG tool). Physician-nurse teams need to collaborate and develop a safe sedation method for those patients that appear to be candidates for moderate sedation. If needed anesthesia should be consulted.

Reference:
1. American College of Physicians. (2013). *Sleep apnea*. Retrieved from http://www.acponline.org/patients_families/diseases_conditions/sleep_apnea/
2. The Durham VAMC Patient Safety Center of Inquiry (PSCI). (2011, march 29). Moderate sedation toolkit for non-anesthesiologists. Retrieved from http://www.patientsafety.gov/pubs.html
3. ESLINGER, M. R. (n.d.). Moderate sedation certification. Retrieved from www.sedationcertification.com
4. *SedationFacts.org*. Sleep Apnea and other Sedation Complications. September 29,2008. http://sedation.sgna.org
5. Urman, Richard D. and Kaye, Alan D. Moderate and Deep Sedation in Clinical Practice. Cambridge University Press, 2012.

Chronic Obstructive Pulmonary Disease (COPD)

Chronic Obstructive Pulmonary Disease (COPD) is the most common lung disease. It is characterized by a progressive inflammation and/or destruction of the parenchyma (bronchioles, bronchi, blood vessels, interstitium, and alveoli), resulting in increased resistance of expiratory gas flow and poor gas exchange. COPD is frequently found in individuals who smoke and those with chronic emphysema or bronchitis [1][12]. According to the National Heart, Lung, and Blood Institute, there are approximately 12 million individuals in the United States diagnosed with Chronic Obstructive Pulmonary Disease, and about another 12 million individuals who are unaware they have this disease. The highest prevalence of COPD cases appears to be those living in and around the Ohio and lower Mississippi Rivers [3] [9].

COPD, ultimately leads to hypoxemia and hypercapnia of the individual affected, making them high risk patients to moderately sedate. Sedation medications can cause severe respiratory depression by compromising the chronic hypercarbia system of the patient. Other risks from the administration of sedation include[1]:

- Hypoventilation
- Hypercapnia
- Bronchospasms
- Oversedation

Considerations and recommendations for sedating the COPD patient [4][5][6][7][8][10][11]:

- Treat any reversible respiratory conditions or exacerbations prior to sedation and procedure with bronchodilators, steroids and/or antibiotics.

- Avoid lying flat, the supine position impairs chest wall muscle function and decreases functional residual capacity and oxygenation.

- Provide supplemental oxygen as needed.

- Have reversal agents, emergency airway and equipment ready.

- When administering sedative medication titrate slowly and give in smaller doses.

- Recommend the administration of medications that have the least affect on the respiratory system, such as Precedex.

- Avoid using a non-rebreather on COPD patients. Administering oxygen through a non-rebreather mask will cause hyperoxia and may result in intubation of the patient. If high flow oxygen is require the Venturi mask provides 24%-60% oxygen concentrations and is the most appropriate for this population [7][10].

Individuals with COPD are at a higher risk for respiratory complications during moderate sedation due to their already compromised respiratory system. It is essential to assess these patients pre-procedure to ensure that they receive any preventative or reversible medications necessary to decrease their chances of respiratory failure during moderate sedation.

References:

1. A.D.A.M. Medical Encyclopedia. (2011, may). *Chronic obstructive pulmonary disease*. Retrieved from http://www.ncbi.nlm.nih.gov/pubmedhealth/PMH0001153/
2. American Society of Anesthesiologists. Practice Guidelines for the Perioperative Management of Patients with Obstructive Sleep Apnea. Anesthesiology. 2006;104:1081-93
3. Center for Disease Control and Prevention. (2013, April). *Chronic obstructive pulmonary disease*. Retrieved from http://www.cdc.gov/copd/data.htm
4. The Durham VAMC Patient Safety Center of Inquiry (PSCI). (2011, march 29). Moderate sedation toolkit for non-anesthesiologists. Retrieved from http://www.patientsafety.gov/pubs.html
5. ESLINGER, M. R. (n.d.). Moderate sedation certification. Retrieved from www.sedationcertification.com

6. The joint commission. (2012). Retrieved from http://www.jointcommission.org
7. Kelly, C. & Riches, A. (2008, January 21). Best practice: Emergency oxygen for respiratory patients. *Nursing Times.net*, Retrieved from http://www.nursingtimes.net/nursing-practice/clinical-zones/respiratory/best-practice-emergency-oxygen-for-respiratory-patients/524416.article
8. Kost, M. (2004). Moderate sedation/analgesia. (2nd ed.). St. Louis: Saunders.
9. National Heart, Lung, and Blood Institute. (n.d.). *Chronic obstructive pulmonary disease*. Retrieved from http://www.nhlbi.nih.gov/health/public/lung/copd/campaign-materials/html/copd-atrisk.htm
10. Sabo, M (2013) What is a non-rebreather mask? http://www.livestrong.com/article/191059-what-is-a-non-rebreather-mask/#ixzz2UhAZQHDL
11. *SedationFacts.org*. Sleep Apnea and other Sedation Complications. September 29,2008. http://sedation.sgna.org
12. Urman, Richard D. and Kaye, Alan D. Moderate and Deep Sedation in Clinical Practice. Cambridge University Press, 2012.

Chronic Opioid use
Methadone
Suboxone
Substance Abuse

Brief History of an Epidemic

Treatment of pain with Opioids has been around since the Sumerians circa 4000 B.C. Homer, Hippocrates, and Claudius Galen all recommended opium for whatever ailed the sick. It wasn't until the 19th century that the addiction to Opioids became apparent. In 1875 the first U. S Laws on regulation of Opioids were made, putting a halt to Opioid abuse. During the 1990's physicians only prescribed pain medications if the patient was terminally ill or had cancer. By 2002, physicians quickly became greatly criticized by the public and media on this practice. The New York Times wrote an article stating that 30 million Americans suffer from chronic pain. In the article, the Times stated, that doctors are reluctant to prescribe pain medications leaving approximately 80% of those with chronic pain untreated. Public statements such as the Times, reflected greatly on images of physicians. With pain management being an epidemic the American Pain Society and the American Academy of Pain Medicine developed chronic pain guidelines. Soon after the Veteran Affairs hospital (VA) named Pain as the 5th vital sign in order to help recognize and treat pain. In 1995 Oxycotin was released for use and prescription pain killers' sales rose 90% from 1997 to 2005.

The National Institute on Drug Abuse (NIDA) reported that in 2010, 7 million people in the United States were using prescription drugs non-medically [4]. These drugs included pain relievers, tranquilizers, stimulants and sedatives. Pain Relievers are, however, the most abused prescription drug. The states with the highest prescription pain medication use are the following per 2011 CDC [22]:

Box 20	U.S States with Highest Pain Medication Use	
	Maine	Florida
	Tennessee	Kentucky
	Arkansas	Nevada
	Oregon	Washington
	West Virginia	Alabama
	Oklahoma	

Patients taking Opioids

Patients that are chronic opioid users or abusers are high risk and difficult to moderately sedate for several reasons. The first reason is that those patients who use opioids for long periods of time, tend to have enhanced pain sensitivity and become less tolerant to pain, which leads to a higher dose of opioids during a procedure than what a healthy normal adult would need [25].

Another reason this population may be high risk or difficult to moderately sedate includes the use of polypharmacy. There are often times that patients may be walking around with xanax, oxycotin and other medications on board. For both these reasons chronic opioid users can experience life-threatening respiratory depression during moderate sedation. Respiratory depression is the most significant serious adverse event risk with all opioid agonists and can result in death. Increased respiratory depression is also seen in the elderly, critically ill, debilitated patients, and in COPD populations, particularly when opioids are given in combination with other agents that depress respiratory drive or consciousness. To reduce the risk of respiratory depression, appropriate dosing and titration are necessary [20].

Suggestions and Considerations [13][21]

- Review patients home medications
- Evaluate pain status and level of comfort
- Consider a multimodal pain management approach. The administration of intravenous Acetaminophen or NSAIDS analgesics 30 mins to 1 hr prior to the procedure has shown to help manage pain during and after procedures.

Numerous studies have shown that multimodal treatment plans can produce considerable opioid dose sparing effects. With the addition of reducing opioid administration and minimizing opioid related adverse effects this multi-modal approach can improve pain relief, increase patient satisfaction and reduce health care costs [21].

- Anxiety is often a precursor as to how much pain one experiences. A more frequent administration of versed may be needed to help co-induce the patient.

- Other drugs to consider if allowed by state board and institution are Ketamine and Precedex, both have little effect on the respiratory system.

- Be sure to titrate medications slowly, some patients may require a lot of analgesics while others may need very little. Be vigilant about vital signs especially respiratory. Stop procedure if patient does not appear to be tolerating the moderate sedation plan. Anesthesia services may meet the patients needs better.

Methadone & Suboxone

If you happen to reside in one of the states with the highest drug and prescription pain medication abuse, then you may find that your state has a higher number of individuals on methadone or Suboxone as well. This of course makes since considering the U.S is fighting to decrease the amount of drug abuse by increasing access to substance abuse treatment centers. Other implications for the rise in the administration of methadone and subutex are pain control. Some studies have shown that methadone and subutex may be better at controlling pain than the typical opioids such as morphine, dilaudid, and oxycotin. In 2009 the CDC, stated that more than 4 million methadone prescriptions alone were written for pain. Both of these medications can , however, make it more challenging to control pain and anxiety during a procedure with moderate sedation [19][23].

There are no specific standards or regimens that guide a moderate sedation team in the most appropriate treatment for this particular population. Some pain management physicians may suggest ketamine, propofol and/or general anesthesia for these patients. However with the growing number of patients waiting for their procedures to be performed, and the increasing of anesthesiologists shortage, it is hard to accommodate our patients. Because demand is greater than supply, more and more moderate sedation nurses and their privilege physicians are finding themselves administering moderate sedation to this population.

Both methadone and buprenorphine (Suboxone) are synthetic opioids, used mainly for the treatment of opioid dependency, abuse and or addiction, but methadone can be sometimes be used for pain control as well [4].

Methadone

Methadone is a full opiate agonist. This means that methadone will give the user the same pain relief or feel as an endorphin without the euphoria or "High" feeling as a prescription pain killer. The half life methadone is approximately 15-60 hrs with a mean of 22 hrs.

Considerations for moderatly sedating a methadone patient [13][23]:

- Screen and monitor for substance abuse during initial patient interview.
- Use prescription drug monitoring programs to identify patients who are misusing or abusing methadone or other prescription painkillers.
- Monitor patients on high doses of methadone for heart rhythm problems.
- The higher the dose of Methadone, the more likely the mu receptors will be saturated and other opioids like fentanyl will be block from penetrating them. Over saturation of the mu receptors makes other opioids ineffective for pain control.
- This population may benefit from a multimodal approach to pain control rather than giving extensive amounts of opioids. Some multimodal drugs to consider include the administration of: Benadryl, Toradol and/or acetaminophen. Versed in combination with the patients normal dose of methadone can also cause a co-induction response and moderate sedation should result even without the administration of additional opioids. Often times the patient will receive enough pain control from their

- normal dose of methadone that they will not require any additional pain medication. Keep in mind that these methods may be appropriate for places like the ER, Interventional Radiology and Cath labs, but Endo may have to use a different approach such as the administration of precedex or propofol to achieve sedation.
- Like other narcotic medicines, methadone can cause respiratory depression, even long after the pain-relieving effects of the medication wear off.
- Methadone can be particularly risky when used with tranquilizers, benzodiazepines and other opioids. The combination puts these patients at a high risk for respiratory depression.
- Long term use of methadone may require higher doses of opioids to achieve effective analges and sedation.
- Always titrate slowly.

Suboxone

Suboxone is a partial opiate agonist. It contains buprenorphine, a strong analgesic and naloxone, an opiate antagonist. The Buprenorphine in Suboxone takes the place of the opiate the abuser has been misusing by saturating opiate receptors in the brain, keeping them from with drawling or desiring more. The Naloxone that is included in Suboxone keeps the user from injecting and abusing the medication. It is an opiate antagonist that inhibits the effects of opioids such as morphine, codeine, and heroin. Naloxone supposedly stays inactive if used sublingually (under the tongue). However, naloxone can sometimes be found in the user's urine when monitored for compliancy. Suboxone, when crushed and injected, in attempt to be abused by the abuser, most certainly activates the naloxone and causes, immediate withdrawal in an opiate-dependent person [4][17].

Considerations for moderately sedating a patient taking Suboxone [4][17]:
- Screen and monitor for substance abuse during initial patient interview.
- Prescription drug monitoring programs can be used to identify patients who may be misusing or abusing prescription painkillers.

- Note that suboxone like methadone will saturate the mu pain receptors at high doses, such as 24-32mg per day. Saturation of the mu pain receptors will keep other opioids from penetrating making them useless in pain relief.
- Methods to consider for areas such as Interventional radiology, Radiology, Cath lab, and ED, include multi modal pain control approaches. Benadryl, Toradol and/or acetaminophen administration prior to the procedure may prove beneficial. Versed in combination with the patients normal dose of suboxone will cause a co-induction response and moderate sedation should occur even without the administration of additional opioids. Often times the patient will receive enough pain control from their normal dose of suboxone they may not require any additional pain medications.
- The elimination half-life of buprenorphine is 20–73 hours.
- Suboxone may increase the effects of other drugs that cause drowsiness, including antidepressants, muscle relaxants, antihistamines, sedatives, other pain relievers, anxiety medicines, and alcohol.
- Buprenorphine can slow your breathing and when mixed with a benzodiazepine the patient becomes at risk for respiratory depression.

Drug & ETOH abuse

ETOH

It is important to ask patients what their alcohol intake is during the pre-assessment phase. Patients that are chronic alcohol consumers generally have multisystem disease. Chronic alcoholism may lead to cirrhosis, elevated liver enzymes, esophageal varies, electrolyte disturbances and etc. All these diseases may make your patient difficult to sedate. In fact chronic alcohol consumers generally require more sedation than the typical patient due to the constant stimulation of the cytochrome p-450 system [13]. The cytochrome P-450 system is a group of enzymes that uses iron to oxidize things. it is part of the body's strategy to dispose of potentially harmful substances by making them more water-soluble . Metabolic clearance of drugs is one function of CYP [8].

However chronic alcohol metabolism in the liver by the enzyme cytochrome P450 2E1 (CYP2E1) creates a harmful condition known as oxidative stress, leading to tissue damage [18].

Even though the chronic alcohol users usually require a higher dose or more frequent dose of sedation to become moderately sedated they also have the issue of prolonged sedation recovery [13]. It is important to keep in mind that the damage liver may require more or higher doses of sedation to be effective but the same liver has a hard time clearing those medications given during a procedure.

What to do if suspected of consuming the day of procedure

A patient with acute alcohol consumption is entirely different than a chronic alcohol user. The sedation requirement would be much less, assuming the patient does not have multisystem disease and liver damage [13].

Regardless of whether your patient is a chronic or acute alcohol consumer, the patient needs to avoid alcohol consumption the night before and /or the day of the procedure [5]. If the patient is suspected of consuming alcohol, a blood alcohol serum level should be performed (with the patient's permission.)If the patient refuses to give permission and/ or is positive for alcohol in the blood stream, then cancelation of the procedure is warranted. Explain to the patient that proceeding on would put the patient in unnecessary harm for aspiration and potentially over-sedation [13].

Consideration for patients who consume alcohol:

- Reschedule the procedure if patient is suspected of consuming alcohol the day of the procedure via evidence of a positive blood alcohol serum for alcohol and /or refuses to have blood drawn for blood alcohol level.

- These patients may require a higher and/or more frequent dose of moderate sedation.

- The patient may take longer to recover than a patient who does not consume alcohol on a daily basis.

- Advise patient not to drink alcohol for 24 hours after receiving conscious sedation.

Prescription and illicit Stimulants

Prescription

A patient using prescription amphetamines are predispose to cardiac dysrhythmias, tachycardia, and cardiac conduction complications. Common prescription stimulants that are usually used are for weight loss, attention deficit disorders, and narcolepsy (see box 21) Despite the prescription name, it is strongly suggested that patients on amphetamines receive a baseline 12-lead EKG and labs associated with cardiac conduction before moderate sedation is provided [2][13].

Box 21	Common Prescription Amphetamines		
Adderall	Ritalin	Provigil	Procentra
Adipex	Concerta	Nuvigil	Dextrostat
Dexedrine	Xyrem	Mthylin	

Resource: Amphetamine, http://www.drugs.com/ingredient/amphetamine.html

Illicit Stimulants

Ecstasy

Ecstasy and cocaine are two types of illicit stimulants commonly used. Ecstasy was first introduce in the mid 1980's and is primarily used as a party drug because of its yielding energizing effect and enhanced pleasure from tactile experiences. The onset of ecstasy is approximately 20 to 45 mins after administration. The affects can last up to 6 hrs. Ecstasy is a synthetic drug that chemically resembles the combination of methamphetamine and the hallucinogen mescaline [10][13]. Mood, aggression, sexual activity, sleep, and sensitivity to pain are all primarily affected by ecstasy [10].

Other physiological side effects include tachycardia, tachypnea, altered mental status, profuse sweating, and hyperthermia.

Complications associated with ecstasy include [10]:

- In high doses, Ecstasy can hinder the body's ability to regulate temperature causing hyperthermia. If not treated the liver, kidney, and cardiovascular system may fail. If condition goes un-treated death may occur.

Considerations for a patient that has recently used Ecstasy [10]:

- In the pre-assessment phase illicit drug use questions should be inquired about.

- If patient appears symptomatic of using an illicit drug on the day of procedure, a drug screen should be ordered. If patient is positive for drug use then they are to be rescheduled for another time and should be seen in the emergency department for presenting symptomatology.

Cocaine

Cocaine is a crystalline tropane alkaloid, derived from the coca plant native to South America. The natives of South America mountains used the leaves as stimulants to help with breathing and stamina while working. In the United States it was first synthesized in 1855 and by 1880 it was recognized in the medical field. At this time cocaine's biggest advocate was the world famous psychologist Sigmund Freud. Freud promoted cocaine as a safe and useful tonic for depression and sexual impotence. By 1886 cocaine made its way as an ingredient in the well-known soda, Coca Cola. It was the euphoric and energizing effect of cocaine that made Coca Cola the most popular soft drink in history. From the 1850's to the 1900's life was good. All social classes were utilizing cocaine in tonics, elixirs and wines. Thomas Edison used cocaine along with many other famous individuals, especially actors and actresses. Cocaine made its way into Hollywood and was a mainstay in the silent film industry. It wasn't until years later that the dangers of drugs like cocaine and opium were made apparent [11].

Cocaine is popular because it causes a euphoric effect with increased energy, reduced fatigue and heightens alertness. Snorting, injecting, and smoking are the common routes of administration. The pleasurable effects of cocaine only last for a short time, 5-30 minutes depending on route of administration, there is a repeated need to keep administering [6].

Common effects seen after cocaine administration include [6]:
- Users may be talkative, extraverted, and have a loss of appetite or need for sleep.
- Some users report feelings of restlessness, irritability, and anxiety.
- Other physical effects of cocaine include constricted blood vessels, dilated pupils, and elevated temperature, heart rate, and blood pressure.

Complications of cocaine administration [13]:
- Negative inotropic and chronotropic effects on the heart muscles.
- Hypertension, myocardial ischemia and/or infarction, dysrhythmias, cerebral hemorrhaging and seizures.

Considerations for patients that use cocaine include [13]:
- During the pre-procedure phase ask about illicit drug use.
- If patient has a history of illicit drug use, perform a baseline ECG prior to the procedure and sedation. An ECG can confirm any evidence of a silent cardiac ischemia episode up to 6 wks after the last administration of cocaine.
- Patients that have used cocaine recently should have their procedure and sedation postponed for 24-48hrs.
- A thorough assessment of the patient's nasal mucosa and structure needs to be performed.
- cocaine induced asthma and other cocaine induce pulmonary complications need to be assessed. A chest x-ray prior to procedure may be needed to rule out any pulmonary related issues.
- Ketamine should be avoided due to its ability to potentiate the cardiovascular toxicity of cocaine.
- The use of naloxone (Narcan) may exaggerate the actions of cocaine.

Downers: Benzodiazepines and Marijuana

Benzodiazepines

Benzodiazepines are widely prescribed for their therapeutic efficacy in reducing anxiety, inducing sleep and suppressing panic symptoms. Benzodiazepines are also commonly prescribed for other reasons as well, such as muscle spasticity, convulsive disorders, pre-surgical sedation, involuntary movement disorders, and detoxification from alcohol and other substances. Although benzodiazepines are very beneficial for multiple conditions chronic use leads to cross tolerance and addiction. Therefore individuals that use benzodiazepines for long periods of times are sometimes difficult to moderately sedate [1].

Listed among the top 100 of most commonly prescribed benzodiazepines include:
- alprazolam (Xanax),
- clonazepam (Klonopin),
- diazepam (Valium)
- and lorazepam (Ativan)

Consideration for patients with chronic benzodiazepine use:
- Benadryl is a nice compliment to an opioid and benzodiazepine mix. Studies have shown that the addition of Benadryl adds a synergistic effect for sedating patients [7].

Marijuana

Marijuana or cannabis comes from the hemp plant known to grow wild in Central and South Asia. The Chinese have documented its use for medical reason as early as 2737 B.C. Marijuana made its way from China to India, South Africa and then Europe by 500 A.D. In 1545 the Spanish brought marijuana to the new world and by 1611 it had infiltrated Jamestown. Here it was grown as a commercial crop along aside the tobacco plant. The use for it at this time was solely to provide fiber [12]. The American government encouraged the growth of the hemp plant in the 17th century for the manufacture of rope, sails, and clothing [12][16]. By 1890 marijuana's value plummeted while cotton became the next big crop. Marijuana was used as an ingredient in some medications but opium and cocaine where the biggest fad to cure alignments. The re-emergence of marijuana is thought to be brought on by the end of the Mexican Revolution of 1910 and/or the Prohibition, this time for recreational use [12][16]. Around the 1850's to 1940's marijuana was again used as medicinal reasons but by the 1930's the U.S. Federal Bureau of Narcotics thought marijuana was an addicting drug that would gateway individuals into narcotic addiction [12][16].

Today Marijuana is considered a psychoactive drug that is used both for medical and recreational use.

Common medicinal uses include but are not limited to [14]:
- Glaucoma
- Anorexia
- Pain

- Multiple sclerosis
- Kidney transplant
- Cancer

Like other medications marijuana has side effects and adverse effects when mixed with other drugs.

Some side effects of marijuana include [9][13][14]:

- heart arrhythmias and blood pressure problems
- lung problems such as pulmonary edema
- impaired mental functioning
- panic reactions
- hallucinations & flashbacks
- sleepiness
- increased appetite

Considerations for patients who use marijuana [9][13][14]:

- During the pre-procedure phase patients should be interviewed on their history, use, and frequency of illicit drug use.
- Because marijuana has over 286 different chemicals it can cause excessive sedation if combined with medications used during and after procedures and/or surgery.
- The tetrahydrocannabinol (THC), one chemical in marijuana, can alone affect the acetylcholine, cardiovascular, respiratory and heat regulating systems in the body.
- Any drug that causes respiratory or cardiac depression may be augmented by cannabis.
- **It is recommended that marijuana users refrain from surgery and/or procedures that will include sedation for at least 2 weeks.** This is due to marijuana's effects on the central nervous system. Marijuana is known to slow the central nervous system too much when combined with anesthesia putting the patient at unnecessary risks for sedation complications.

Summary

The pre-procedure phase plays a key part in the assessment of the patient's social history. Many patients may not confess to any illicit or substance use due to fear of being reported or ashamed.

However, assure them that you only wish for them to have a safe and uncomplicated procedure. Educate the patient as well on the possibility of life threatening complications from illicit drug or substance use when combined with sedation. Lastly, this population of patients may need additional support that includes psychiatric and social services.

Reference:
1. Addiction: Part I. Benzodiazepines—Side Effects, Abuse Risk and Alternatives, LANCE P. LONGO, M.D., BRIAN JOHNSON *Am Fam Physician.* 2000 Apr 1;61(7):2121-2128.
2. *Amphetamine.* (n.d.). Retrieved from http://www.drugs.com/ingredient/amphetamine.html
3. Byrne, A., Hallian, R., Watson, R., & Wodak, A. (2005). Methadone vs. buprenorphine. *British Journal of General Practice, 55,* 516. doi: PMC1472782
4. Buprenorphine. (n.d) Retrieved from http://www.drugs.com/mtm/buprenorphine-injection.html#xkAB9aKvU0JIKZ71.99
5. Clinical Center National Institute of Health, conscious sedation for adults. (2007). Retrieved from http://www.cc.nih.gov/ccc/patient_education/pepubs/consed.pdf
6. *Cocaine.* (n.d.). Retrieved from , http://www.drugs.com/cocaine.html
7. Contending with sedation challenges. (2006, April 1). *Endo Nurse,* Retrieved from http://www.endonurse.com/articles/2006/04/contending-with-sedation-challenges.aspx
8. Davis, N. (2006). *Cytochrome p450.* Retrieved from http://anaesthetist.com/physiol/basics/metabol/cyp/Findex.htm
9. Dickerson, S. J. (1980). Cannabis and its effect on anesthesia. *Journal of the American Association of Nurse Anesthetists,* 526-528.
10. *Ecstasy, what is ecstasy.* (n.d.). Retrieved from http://www.drugs.com/ecstasy.html
11. *History of cocaine.* (n.d.). Retrieved from http://www.narconon.org/drug-information/cocaine-history.html

12. *History of marijuana.* (n.d.). Retrieved from http://www.narconon.org/drug-information/marijuana-history.html
13. Kost, M. CRNA, MS, Forren, J. RN, MS, CPAN, FAAN. Administration of Moderate Sedation/Analgesia. 9/7/2012, http://ce.nurse.com/ce159-60/administration-of-moderate-sedationanalgesia/
14. *Marijuana*. (2009). Retrieved from http://www.webmd.com/vitamins-supplements/ingredientmono-947-MARIJUANA.aspx?activeIngredientId=947&activeIngredientName=MARIJUANA
15. *Marijuana.* (2013). Retrieved from http://www.rxlist.com/script/main/art.asp?articlekey=96910&pf=3&page2
16. *Marijuana timeline.* (n.d.). Retrieved from http://www.pbs.org/wgbh/pages/frontline/shows/dope/etc/cron.hml
17. *Methadone vs. suboxone.* (n.d.). Retrieved from http://www.diffen.com/difference/Methadone_vs_Suboxone
18. National Institute of Alcohol Abuse and Alcoholism, Alcohol Metabolism's Damaging Effects on the Cell, A Focus on Reactive Oxygen Generation by the Enzyme Cytochrome P450 2E1, by Dennis R. Koop, Ph.D. http://pubs.niaaa.nih.gov/publications/arh294/274-280.htm
19. *NIH, topics in brief: Prescription drug.* (n.d.). Retrieved from http://www.drugabuse.gov/publications/topics-in-brief/prescription-drug-abuse
20. *Partners against pain, general safety information on opioid analgesics.* (n.d.). Retrieved from http://www.partnersagainstpain.com/hcp/pain-assessment/opioid-analgesics-safety.aspx
21. Pasero, C., & Stannard, D. (2012). The role of intravenous acetaminophen in acute pain management. *Pain Management Nursing, 13*(2), 107-124. Retrieved from www.medscape.com

22. Prescription painkiller: Overdoses in the U.S. (2011, November). *Center for disease control*, Retrieved from http://www.cdc.gov/VitalSigns/PainkillerOverdoses/
23. Prescription painkiller overdoses use and abuse of methadone as a painkiller. (2012, July). *CDC Vital Signs*, Retrieved from http://www.cdc.gov/vitalsigns/MethadoneOverdoses/
24. The Society of Gastroenterology Nurses and Associates http://sedation.sgna.org
25. Streltzer, J. (2001). Pain management in the opioid-dependent patient. *Current Psychiatry Reports*, 3(6), 489-496.

Urman, Richard D. and Kaye, Alan D. Moderate and Deep Sedation in Clinical Practice. Cambridge University Press, 2012.

Chapter 9
Challenging Circumstances

As sedation nurse, you may already know that sedation cases do not sometimes go as smoothly as they could have. Often times preventive measures could have been applied to make these cases less complicated. There are also times when a nurse must use his or her professional judgment either for rescue, ethics, or advocacy in sedating a patient. This chapter consists of case scenarios and Q&A addressing complex challenges.

Scenario 1: 1,000cc of Oral Contrast

John is a 56yr white male requiring a ct guided abscess drain in the abdomen. He has a diagnosis of GERD, reflux, HTN, DMII, and morbid obesity. His labs are within normal limits and vital signs are all stable:

> hrt= 66
> b/p= 130/60
> O2 sat= 94% on RA
> resp= 20

The physician performing the procedure is credentialed in moderate sedation. In order for the physician to perform the procedure the patient must drink 1,000cc of contrast so that bowel is visualized on the scan. After finishing the contrast the patient is called to the ct procedure room for the procedure to begin. Upon arrival of the patient the sedation nurse performs her assessment. she realizes that the patient has drank contrast recently, therefore has not been NPO according to ASA guidelines.

Question: What should the nurse do?

1. Moderately Sedate the patient as ordered
2. Consult Anesthesiologist expert opinion
3. Contact manager
4. Refuse to participate in case

Discussion:

This can be a very difficult position for a nurse to be in. NPO guidelines rarely mention amount of fluid and oral contrast.

> As, per a study conducted in 2010, on Gastric emptying time of oral contrast material in children and adolescents undergoing abdominal computed tomography, it concluded that a patient should be NPO for 3hrs after ingesting oral contrast [1]

The nurse understands that the patient needs the biopsy and the physician needs the patient to consume the contrast so he does not injure bowel while performing the biopsy. The nurse believes that although the procedure and contrast consumption are necessary, the patient is at risk for aspiration due to volume of contrast, loss of gag reflex from sedation, supine position, and history of GERD and Reflux.

Suggestions:

1. Explain to the physician that you are teamed with, that you understand the importance of the procedure, however you do not feel comfortable sedating a patient who has recently consumed 1,000cc of contrast. Suggest to the physician perhaps performing the procedure without sedation but with local anesthesia and minimal opioids for comfort.

2. Suggest to the physician that you feel this is beyond your scope of practice and anesthesia services may need consulted to protect the patients airway.

3. Consult with an anesthesiologist, after all they are doctors of sedation and analgesia. They may be able to help you offer alternative solutions.

4. If necessary the physician can administer the moderate sedation while the nurse monitors the patient. The physician however needs to explain to the patient the risks associated with administering sedation without being NPO. The physician also needs to document a rationale in the patients chart. See ASA Sedation Model Policy.

> **ASA Sedation Model Policy**
> Certain radiological procedures require the administration of oral fluids in conjunction with sedation and analgesia. Risk of aspiration during these procedures must be weighed against the benefits of sedation and analgesia. Patients undergoing these types of procedures must be informed of risks. The following is not a recommendation but a suggestion: In the event that the NPO requirements are adjusted, the credentialed physician may administer moderate sedation with operating monitoring personnel and appropriate documentation to include rationale must be included in the medical record [8].

5. Communicate with your manager, make them aware of the specialized case. Also communicate that a resolution was able to be made or not. If needed communicate that patient safety is a concern and the procedure requires an advanced healthcare provider to sedate and monitor the patient.

Scenario 2: Vomiting

An 86yr African American male inpatient has been called to an Interventional Radiology (IR) Suite for a Percutanous Transhepatic Cholangiogram and drain placement. The patient has a tumor blocking the bile duct and has been experiencing nausea most of the day. The IR nurse gather report from the floor nurse:

> V/S stable
> GCS =15
> MIVF via 20g in right hand infusing
> Patient vomited less than 100cc 2hrs ago and has received 4mg of Zofran immediately after.
> Patient has been NPO for 8hrs

Upon arrival the IR nurse performs a quick assessment of the patients status. Patient states that he still feels nausea. The doctor performing the procedure is consulted and orders for Zofran 8mg IVP now were verbalized. The medication is administered by the IR nurse and the patient vomits 100cc in a basin. The charge nurse is contacted by the IR nurse stating the that patient is not a good candidate for moderate sedation and to begin working on alternatives so procedure can be performed. The IR nurse informs the physician that the patient is not an appropriate candidate for moderate sedation at this time. The physician orders for the nurse to wait 15mins then if no vomiting occurs move patient to procedure table and have him prepped for procedure. 15minutes pass and the patient is transferred to the procedure table with the assistance of radiology technologists and the nurse. The nurse begins to connect the required monitoring equipment when patient projectile vomits green black emesis across the room. The physician is informed of status and orders more Zofran. The nurse feels that the patient is unstable for procedure to continue and contacts the charge nurse and management with the suggestion of anesthesia services. The charge nurse has already contacted anesthesia services and has confirmed that an anesthesia provider can provide services in 30 min. The charge nurse verbalizes to manager and physician that anesthesia services are available to perform procedure. The physician is still not willing to consider anesthesia services at this time. Manager is then contacted with status and approaches physician.

After the department manager and physician discuss situation, the agreement of the patient receiving sedation and analgesia by anesthesia services has been made.

Anesthesia arrives and intubates the patient. An OG tube is placed and over 500cc of black/green content is aspirated from stomach. The physician performing the procedure later reported to the department manager that the nurses assessment was appropriate.

Discussion

Did the nurse do the right thing?

Not all cases go as smoothly as planned. Sometimes it is difficult to decide which patients are appropriate for moderate sedation and which patients are not. Is not always black and white, sometimes like the patient in this case, they can be borderline between moderate sedation by a physician-nurse team and requiring anesthesia services.

Because the IR nurse performed a quick assessment of the patient upon arrival to the IR room, she was able to prepare for an preventive measures for vomiting and develop an alternate plan for sedation. The nurse alerted the IR charge nurse that anesthesia services may be needed and informed the physician the patient was still experiencing nausea.

Even though it was difficult to convince the physician that the patient would receive safer care under anesthesia services the nurse gained respect for her decision and planning in the end.

What if anesthesia services would have not been available?

> *Performing a good assessment of the patient, providing sound evidence for potential complications, and providing reasonable alternatives will most likely provide you the right support for your decisions.*

What if anesthesia services could not provide services at the time of request? Could another alternative be considered.

There are times when anesthesia services can not accommodate the physician-nurse team and patient because of emergencies. Some institutions have a triage system for anesthesia services. One example is an operating room anesthesia request form. This form asks for the requesting service to list the nature of the case and the status of the case such as Emergent, Stat, routine, etc. Based on the status completed on the card, anesthesia services has to provide their service within in so many hours.

The another consideration for this scenario could be:

- Have the patient return to the floor.

- Have primary service contacted and begin antiemetic therapies, such as, H2 inhibitors, antiemetic medications, and placement of an NG tube placement with intermittent suction.

- Reassess patient's status as a candidate for moderate sedation in an hour.

Scenario 3: Hypotensive

A 56 yr old Asian female, outpatient, has been called to the IR suite for a cerebral angiogram. The IR nurse receives report from the patients floor nurse:

Patient's v/s:
b/p 110/50
hrt 54
resp 22
temp 36.6
O2 sat 92% on room air
Able to lay prone
NPO for 8 hrs

The patient arrives to the IR suite

Consents are verified

H&P verified (ASA2, mallampati =2)

The patient is placed on the procedure table, prepped and draped for the procedure. Time out is completed, physician verbally orders 50mcg of fentanyl and 1 mg of versed before sheath is placed. 5mins pass and physician begins to access groin for sheath placement. Patient begins to scream and holler with local anesthetic. V/S are as follows:

Hrt 50

b/p 90/40 maps in 60's

O2 sat 90% RA

RR 22

The physician verbally orders another 50mcg of fentanyl and 1 mg of Versed. The nurse asks the physician if he can increase the fluid rate to help counter act the side effects of fentanyl's hypotensive properties. The physician agrees. The nurse increases the fluids and gives only 25mcg of fentanyl and 1mg of versed at this time.

The sheath access takes a few minutes and appears to be difficult to place. The patient begins to yell again and is now crying. The physician orders another 50mcg of fentanyl and 1 mg of versed. However the nurse checks the next set of vital signs before administering the ordered dose. VS are as follows:

Hrt 50
b/p 80/40 map in 50's
O2 sat 92%
RR 24

The nurse verbalizes to the physician the current VS. The physician, however wants the dose given anyhow. The nurse states that he does not feel comfortable in administrating another dose at this time due to the current b/p. The physician screams to administer the dose. The nurse turns to the patient and begins to gently touch her forehead and explains that her blood pressure is to low at this time to administer another dose. The nurse begins to ask the patient questions on where she is from and how many kids does she have while continuing to gently stroke her forehead.

The patient appears to have started to relax and the physician places the sheath.

Discussion

It is difficult to see patients in pain- even for physicians. It is also difficult to control a patient's pain if their physiological responses to medications are obtuse. The patient in this scenario may have been experiencing heightened anxiety from not knowing what to exactly to expect during the procedure even though she had signed the consents. It is best to verbalize everything being done while setting up for the procedure and prepping the patient. Fear comes from the unknown. The difficulty of the sheath placement also played a role in pain. Not all patients have stellar anatomy and throbbing pulses. Comforting and distracting the patient while the sheath was placed was a good alternative to administrating another dose of fentanyl.

Some considerations to think about from this scenario:

- Hydration of the patient prior to procedure.
- Greeting the patient and letting her know everybody's role in the procedure.
- Explaining the steps of prepping to the patient and what she may expect to feel during the procedure.

- The suggestion from the nurse to the physician that maybe more local anesthetic could be administered.

- The nurse asking for a little more time for the fentanyl and versed to take effect before starting the sheath placement.

- And perhaps the administration of more versed.

Scenario 4: Supra-Ventricular Tachycardia (SVT)

A 68yr old white male with a history of end stage renal disease, GERD, hypertension, and DM II is scheduled for an outpatient Tunneled Cuff Catheter (TCC) placement for dialysis.

He has been transported from the same day surgical care area to the interventional radiology suite.

The intra-procedure nurse receives report from the same day care pre-procedure nurse. The patients has been NPO x8 hrs, VS are within normal limits, antibiotics were given, patient voided, consents in the chart, and a recent EKG is in the chart showing a normal rhythm.

The patient is moved to the procedure table, cardiopulmonary devices connected and monitored q 5mins. Patient introduced to staff, prepping begins, physician in room and orders first dose of moderate sedation. Pt given 50mcg fentanyl and 1mg versed. Prep completed, physician gowned, all appropriate persons in room, and time out initiated.

During the procedure the nurse notices that the patient begins to have some dysrhythmias. She informs the physician and the physician states "OK, my wire is tickling the heart". The nurse assesses the patient and b/p. The patient is arousable but unable to keep eyes open long enough to follow commands. The blood pressure, respirations, and O2 sat are within normal limits. The nurse then hears an increase in heart rate from the pulse ox device. The patient's rhythm has increased to 180bpm and the nurse believes the patient is experiencing SVT. The nurse informs the physician of the current change in heart rate, while simultaneously assessing LOC, vital signs, and applies O2 for cardiac support. The nurse states that although the patient is currently stable, she is no longer comfortable with the current condition of the patient. The nurse at this time suggests to the physician that an EKG and possible cardiology consult be obtained. The physician removes the tunneled catheter and asks a member of the team to page cardiology to the IR suite. The nurse attempts to arouse the patient , but he is unable to be aroused enough to perform commands such as coughing and baring down.

Cardiology services arrive and an EKG is performed. The patient is experiencing SVT. The cardiopulmonary code cart arrives in the room by a member of the staff. The chest pads are placed and the life pack monitor is turned on. Cardiology prepares the adenosine and asks the nurse to administer the medication. Atropine has also been drawn up and is readily available.

The adenosine is pushed and the heart rate decreases to 40bpm and then stabilizes in the 60's. The IR physician asks one of the cardiology physicians to stay as she wishes to attempt the TCC placement with more caution. The physician begins again, the wire is placed and the catheter advances into the SVC. The patient immediately begins to experience stable SVT. The patient is more arousable at this point and is instructed to perform valsalva maneuver. The maneuver is completed and the patient's procedure is aborted at this time.

Discussion

Did the nurse respond appropriately?

Anytime there are devices in and near the heart there are risks for cardiac complications such as dysrhythmias. The nurse was very attentive to the patient. Although the patient might have been sedated deeper than intended, the patient was stable and able to maintain spontaneous ventilation. Communication with the physician was appropriate and professional judgments were respected.

Scenario 5 : On Call

It is around the fall holidays and the cath lab has had a busy day. With two suites and teams working all day, the cath lab wasn't able to complete all the scheduled and emergent cases. One team leaves at 3:30 while the on-call team stays over to finish the cases for the day. At 10pm the cath lab team is finally starting their last case of the day. The radiology technologists and nurse have been working since 7am are feeling tired, hungry and wore down. The last case finishes at 12am and the cath lab team changes and walks to their vehicles.

The cath lab nurse opens his car door, gets in, closes his eyes and lays his head back against the car seat happy that the day is over. As soon as the nurse turns the keys of his vehicle his pager goes off. A emergent MI needing a catheterization has entered the emergency room. The nurse reluctantly goes back inside, enters the cath suite and preps for the patients arrival. He drawls up his fentanyl and versed, receives report from the ED nurse.

The team is ready, the patient arrives, the patient skips his assessment and forgets to look for consents. The patient is transferred to the procedure table and prepped and draped. The time out is initiated and the procedure begins. The physician orders 50mcg of fentanyl IVP for the sheath placement now. The nurse administered what he thinks is fentanyl but after injecting the medication realizes he has injected 1 mg of versed instead. The nurse informs the physician of his mistake and although it was the wrong medication the physician states that it is fine and to pay attention. The physician asks for the nurse to then give 25mcg of fentanyl now. The case finishes and the nurse remembers he forgot to verify the presence of a consent before the procedure. So he looks for the consents but does not see them. He informs the physician and the physician is irate at the cath lab nurse's lack of responsibility.

Before leaving the cath lab nurse realizes that he may not even be able to drive home. He calls his manager and informs the manager that he is very tired and has made several mistakes in the last case that could have cause serious harm to the patient. He states that he can not continue to be on call and asks the manager to call other nurses to cover the call.

Discussion

Did the nurse respond appropriately?

Endoscopy, Cath Lab, and Interventional Radiology nurses take call after hours, on weeknights, weekends, and holidays to cover emergency procedures. The call team works until the cases are finished. Sometimes even if it's greater than 16 hrs.

Excess hours beyond a scheduled shift leads to errors and burn out. Fatigued nurses can not provide high quality, safe patient care. Depending on state labor laws, working over 16hrs in a 24hr period without 8 hrs of rest is prohibited unless, unforeseen emergencies arise, such as bioterrorism, sever weather, and etc occur. Some states include on call in this category but with special circumstances. On call is consider the acceptance of overtime and if you agreed to abide by this expectation at the time of employment then you are not able to refuse call. As of 2009, 15 states had restrictions on overtime and nurses. Check with your state labor law, board of nursing or state attorney general on overtime, fatigue and on call regulations.

A call nurse can and has every right to ask for permission from the manager to rest for 8 hrs after a 16 hr shift, if they feel that continuing will endanger the quality and safety of the patient. A good and reasonable manager will exhaust all necessary attempts to have the nurse's call covered before ever denying permission to rest.

In the event that call can not be covered, then documentation of attempts to advise the facility/manager of the concern needs to be kept on personal record. The documentation should include time, date, and what the conversation entailed (verbalization of fatigue and patient safety concerns). If a serious error does occur from fatigue than there is documentation that a plan for prevention was attempted [1].

The effects of insufficient sleep have been well researched and documented. Lack of sleep or rest has a variety of adverse effects. Despite the wide range of research methodologies and settings the results are similar: Insufficient sleep has been associated with poor cognition, mood alterations, increased safety risks and reduced job performance and motivation.

Working extended hours has been linked to medical error rates. According to studies, medical errors triple after workers perform for over 12.5 hrs of continuous activity [2]. Even airline and trucking industries understand the correlation of rest and safety. Both industries limit the number of hours pilots and truck drivers can fly/drive. They also require a certain number of hours between "flights" or "runs".

Like the airline and trucking industries, The American Society of Peri-Anesthesia Nurses (ASPAN) understands the importance of hours worked and risks associated to the nurse and patient. It is therefore their responsibility to define the practice of peri-anesthesia nursing and promote safe and appropriate care in this type of nursing. Below in box 24 is the position statement on "On Call/Work Schedule" by the ASPAN.

> **Box 24**   **ASPAN position statement**
>   **" On Call/Work Schedule"**[2]
> - The number and length of on call shifts assigned should be coordinated with the number of sustained work hours and provide adequate recuperation periods.
> - There is a plan in place to relieve the on-call nurse in the event that the manager/nurse determines that there is a potential for compromise in the delivery of safe, competent care without fear of reprisal or disciplinary action.

Scenario 6: Moderate Sedation after General Sedation

A 60 yr old Caucasian male with a past medical history of hypertension, acute renal failure, diabetes mellitus 2, and mild mental disability, underwent a lithotripsy procedure at 0900 with general anesthesia. The patient had was administered reversal agents for fentanyl and versed in the PAR/PACU. The patient appears to be back to baseline according to the PAR/PACU nurse and anesthesiologist. An interventional Radiologist was contacted and asked to place bilateral nephrostomy tubes in the patient since the lithotripsy procedure was unsuccessful in breaking up his kidney stones. Jane a moderate sedation nurse paired with the radiologist, does not feel the procedure should be performed today unless anesthesia services will re-sedate the patient. The nurse expresses concern to the radiologist about high risks of complications from moderately sedating the patient after patient has already received general anesthesia. The radiologist tells the nurse that the procedure must be done today and the he is capable of providing moderate sedation under his privileges.

The nurse against her better judgment calls the PACU to receive report on the patient. In report the nurse receives that the patient is awake, VSS and the preparing to be transferred from PACU to his floor bed.

PT Report:

- Alert x4
- VS: HR=62, RR=22, O2 sat =97%, B/P=150/62
- HX: DMII, HTN, ARF, Mild mental disability (consentable)
- Pt received Narcan in OR

Jane reports to radiologist that the patient has received reversal agents in OR. The radiologist states half life on Narcan has exceeded and to have patient transferred to Interventional Radiology (IR) for Nephrostomy tube placement.

The patient arrives to the IR suite and Jane begins her assessment. The patient appears as the PACU nurse reported. The patient was consented for the nephrostomy tubes by the radiologist.

The patient is positioned prone on the procedure table, continuous VS monitoring of HR, RR, O2 sat and B/P is initiated.

The procedure starts and the patient receives his first dose of fentanyl and versed. VS remain stable throughout procedure however the patient's pain appears to be slightly difficult to control. The radiologist is suturing the second nephrostomy tube when the O2 sat alarms. The nurse visualizes that the monitor is displaying 87%. The nurse quickly assess the patient and applies O2 NC 2 LPM. The patient is difficult to arouse and he continues to desaturate after the administration of O2. The nurse is at the patient head and informs the radiologist that the patient appears dusky and unresponsive. Jane places a non-rebreather and states patient needs to be reversed and supine ASAP. The radiologist gives verbal order for reversal agents.

The patient does not appear to respond, the patient continues to desaturate into the 60's, RR=6, B/P 100/50, HR 90. The patient's bed is moved into the room and patient is transferred to bed in supine position. Rescue breathing with Ambu bag is initiated by radiology technologist and the nurse administers another round of reversal agents. There appears to be no response to the second round of reversal agents, the nurse calls for the code team to arrive.

The code team arrives and provides a patent airway with an endotracheal tube. The patient is transferred to PACU for recovery.

Discussion:

Did the nurse respond appropriately? What could have been done differently?

The physician-nurse moderate sedation team should have respect and trust in each others evaluations and assessments of patients physical status. It is sometimes difficult to decide which patients are appropriate candidates for moderate sedation because they hover around the fine line of being acceptable. If there is any doubt anesthesia services are an excellent resource to consult. A thought here too to consider is, if anesthesia services (trained and specialized in anesthesia and analgesia) are not willing to moderately sedate a patient in his/her current condition, then why would a physician-nurse team take the risk.

If anesthesia services are not available to consult think of the following:

- If the patient receive reversal agents in the PACU, then he did not tolerate general anesthesia well.
- If the patient requires bilateral nephrostomy tube placements, then he probably not eliminating urine via his bladder and therefore is not excreting and metabolizing medications well. from his system appropriately. More than likely he will not be able to do the same with moderate sedation medications as well.

Outcomes that could have been done differently:

- The gastroenterologist, radiologist, and anesthesiologist could have collaborated so that the patient would receive continuation of anesthesia during nephrostomy tube placements after the failure of lithotripsy.

Scenario 7: Intent to sedate

A nurse in the emergency room is ordered to give fentanyl 50 mcg IVP and 1 mg of Ativan IVP to a patient that is about to have a chest tube placed. The nurse asks the physician if he has obtained a consent to sedate and how long the patient has been NPO. The physician states that a single dose of fentanyl and versed IVP given together for a chest tube placement is not consider sedation.

The nurse believes that administrating an opioid and benzodiazepine together, for the purposes of a medical procedure or diagnostic exam, is considered an intent to sedate. She expresses to the physician that she would be more than happy to administer an opioid for the anticipation of pain while inserting a chest tube, but does not feel comfortable administrating an opioid and benzodiazepine together without following appropriate guidelines for sedation. The physician becomes very angry and threatens to take corrective action. The nurse states again that she will administer the fentanyl but not the Ativan without following the hospital sedation policies and practices.

The chest tube was placed with the administration of fentanyl IVP only, The patient appeared to tolerate the placement with minimal discomfort.

Discussion:

Did the nurse respond appropriately?

According to Guidelines for the Use of Sedation and General Anesthesia by Dentists *As adopted by the October 2012 ADA House of Delegates,* when the intent is minimal sedation for adults, the appropriate initial dosing of a single enteral (drug administration via the digestion) medication is no more than the maximum recommended dose (MRD) of a drug that can be prescribed for unmonitored home use.

The medications used in this scenario, Ativan and Fentanyl, by themselves are fairly predictable and rarely results in apnea and loss of consciousness, when given in small single doses.

However, whenever given in combination, especially when administered simultaneously (aka Co-induction),they are unpredictable and the loss of consciousness and or apnea may occur.

This particular act is considered co-induction, which is the act of causing a hypnotic state and was coined around 1986. The name was first introduced when unplanned anesthesia was induced by administering a benzodiazepine combined with an opioid by non-anesthetically trained healthcare providers practicing sedation [4].

> ***The definition for Sedation*** *is the reduction of <u>irritability</u> or agitation by administration of <u>sedative</u> drugs, generally <u>to facilitate a medical procedure or diagnostic procedure</u>. Drugs which can be used for sedation include <u>propofol</u>, <u>etomidate</u>, <u>ketamine</u>, <u>fentanyl</u>, and midazolam [3]*

The risks associated with sedation include: Airway obstruction, apnea and hypotension, and require the presence of health professionals who are suitably trained to detect and manage these problems

Summary

It is likely that everyday a moderate sedation nurse will be challenged at least once during his of her shift. Challenges may included various circumstances such as improper consents, the need for anesthesiology, oversedation, adverse medication reactions, procedural complications, and even sleep deprivation. Having the right amount of training and education in moderate sedation administration and rescue interventions is imperative for successful outcomes.

Reference:
1. Legally speaking…..When can you say NO?, Penny S. Brooke ASPRN, MS, JD, Nursing 2013, july 2009, vol 39, # 7 pages 42-46
2. Perianesthesia Nursing: Standards, Practice Recommendations and Interpretive statements, 2012-2014

Chapter 10
Future Trends and Possibilities

The concept of sedation and analgesia has been around for as long as people have been performing surgeries. People have constantly been searching for the perfect combination of medications to dull the senses and induce sleep . It wasn't however until 1846 that a dentist, William Mortan, discovered ether could be used to control pain and sleep of a patients undergoing surgical procedures [12]. During this time the word anesthesia was coined and the practice took fire.

By the 1980s, an increasing demand of procedures requiring sedation and analgesia took place. Anesthesia services could not meet these demands and physicians turned to nurses for the administration of sedation and analgesia [9]. Today moderate sedation continues to be administered outside the operating room for procedures like bronchoscopy endoscopy, cardiac studies, pacemaker placements, drainage tube placements, and biopsies.

The use of moderate sedation physician-nurse teams continues to increase tremendously and will continue to increase in the future for several reasons. The first most driving reason is healthcare reform, followed by the shortage of anesthesiologist and development of newer drugs and technology.

Health Care Reform

Under the Patient Protection and Affordable Care Act (PPCA) payment will be increasingly driven by value based services and purchasing. Medicare and Medicaid will allow payment for the anaesthesia or sedation services of clinicians who are working within their state licensing laws scope of practice and who are appropriately credentialed.

The physician can bill for moderate sedation services provided by the same physician performing the diagnostic or therapeutic service that the sedation supports. The payment for moderate sedation in this manner is just a fraction of the payment for anaesthesia .

Patients who receive deep sedation or general anesthesia require more costly care by an anesthesiologist or nurse anesthetist. So why pay for anesthesia services when it is more cost effective to use a physician-nurse team to provide sedation for the same procedure.

> *Moderate sedation by a trained and credentialed physician-nurse team can reduce the patients hospital charges by $1800-$2400 (dependent on procedure), as opposed to sedation by an anesthesiologist [2][10][14].*

Since the beginning of the reform in 2010, private and commercial healthcare insurance companies have started to take notice in the cost differences and have denied anesthesia services for procedures like endoscopies.

A study in JAMA, Anesthesia Services Used Unnecessarily for GI Endoscopies, found that the number of endoscopy procedures using anesthesia services for deep sedation or general anesthesia had more than doubled between 2003 and 2009. The number of Medicare patients within this group almost doubled, while commercially insured patients almost increased 4-fold. The most notable discovery within the study was that greater than two thirds of patients were considered low risk (ASA of 3 >) for sedation and could have had moderate sedation by a gastroenterologist-nurse team [1].

The attractiveness of anesthesia services by physicians like endoscopist will more than likely fade in the future. It won't be long before Medicare, private and commercial insurers deny anesthesia services on a normal basis for patients who are considered low risk by ASA standards, to sedate by a physician-nurse team. Forced by the hand of value based payment and the upcoming anesthesiologist shortage, it is likely more sophisticated education and technologies will be adopted to support physician-nurse sedation teams in order to better serve patients and physicians.

Anesthesia Provider Shortage

Since 2012 healthcare professions have seen an influx of the aging population requiring healthcare. This influx has led to a greater need for physicians and other healthcare providers. With a large number of patients over the age of fifty, there has been an increase need for procedures and surgeries. The result of this cause a demand for physicians, especially anesthesiologist.

It is anecdotal whether or not the United States is going to face a shortage of anesthesia providers in the near future. Currently there are approximately 40,000 Anesthesiologists (AN), and 39,000 Certified Registered Nurse Anesthetists (CRNA) and student CRNA's practicing in the U.S. A research team from RAND

Health examined anesthesia labor markets in the U.S and found that as of 2007 there was a nationwide shortage of 3,800 AN's and 1,282 CRNA's. The team also projected that in some scenarios shortages will persist until 2020 [4].

The upcoming anesthesia shortage is presumed to be contributed to several causes. The increase in market and the shrinking of supply is most likely the biggest contributor. The number of procedures requiring anesthesia services outside of the OR, such as MRI, Endoscopy, ambulatory surgical centers, and office based anesthesia is outstripping the supply of anesthesiologist. Other reasons include the increase of baby-boomers who will increase the Medicare population, the retirement of aging anesthesiologists, and little recruitment into anesthesia programs [8].

As a result of the projected deficit of anesthesia services, several events may take place. If no interventions are made to address the greater demand versus supply, then patients will be waiting longer than necessary for surgical procedures and preventable death may occur. The second event that is likely to occur is the increase in use of moderate sedation physician-nurse teams. Anesthesia in this instance will be reserved for high risk surgical procedures. With the shift in care by providers it is also expected that patients receiving moderate sedation by physician-nurse teams will have more complex morbities than today.

With the possible influx in complex morbid patients sedated by physician-nurse teams there has to be accommodations made to safely sedate these types of patients. There will need to be required advanced training and education, the development of new drugs with fewer side effects and/ or advanced monitoring systems to better control drugs currently being utilized.

Newer Drugs & Technology

The process of continual improvement for safe delivery of moderate sedation will open new doors to technology and medications. As opposed to the 1980's moderate sedation now has a good number of short acting drugs available. Although the medications currently being used are effective at achieving the goals and objectives of moderate sedation, they still posse adverse reactions and controversies. In an effort to tackle these matters and improve sedation regimens, alternative pharmaceuticals and delivery methods are being explored. Currently under review by the FDA, are new agents as well as expanded applications for existing ones like precedex are being explored. On the delivery side, a computer-assisted personalized sedation (CAPS) system, Patient controlled sedation/analgesia (PSCSA) and target-controlled infusion (TCI) are examples of possible innovative approaches to sedation administration.

Precedex (Dexmedetomidine)

Precedex, a selective alpha-2-andrenoceptor agonist, is a newer sedative that has moved into the moderate sedation arena. The greatest feature about this medication is that it is a cooperative sedation. Meaning it has both sedative and analgesic effects without respiratory depression. Deeper levels of sedation can be achieved while preserving respiratory functions [15].

It wasn't until 2008, that precedex was approved for the use of procedural sedation outside the OR and ICU. Today it is often seen utilized for procedural sedation in adults and children undergoing cardiac, interventional, and endoscopic procedures. It also does not appear to be restricted by physician-nurse teams use.

> *In a study measuring versed vs. precedex in the sedation of patients requiring upper endoscopies, precedex performed effectively and safely as versed. Precedex was also found superior with regard to gagging, rate of side effects and endoscopist satisfaction. The study concluded that precedex may be a good alternative to midazolam in sedating patients [5].*

Although precedex is superior in that is preserves respiratory function it still has a considerable side effect. The most profound adverse effect appears to effect the vasovagal response, causing bradycardia and hypotension [15].

The discovery for a medication with the best sedative and analgesic properties with the least amount of adverse events, will always be the ultimate goal. But until then continual improvement for safe administration of sedation will likely advance.

Patient controlled sedation/analgesia (PSCSA) and Computer assisted personalized sedation (CAPS) [15]

Controlling sedation without over sedation

The debate has now raged on for years whether drugs like Propofol can be safely administration by a physician-nurse team. Propofol can be dangerous in untrained hands. It is unpredictable, dosing and titration is variable, and it is based on the patient's response and tolerance to the drug. As quality improvement for patient safety continues advancements in the administration for sedation are currently being discovered.

In the attempt to provide safe administration of medications like propofol new technology/methods have emerged. Patient and computer controlled devices/methods, are two developments that can control sedation administration.

Patient controlled sedation/analgesia (PSCSA)

PSCSA is a innovative sedation administration delivery method that resembles today's patient controlled analgesia (PCA) machines. This technique allows the patient to directly control the amount of his or her own sedation and sedation level. Similar to the PCA the PSCSA has many of the same features. The PSCSA has a predetermined infusion rate, bolus mode and lockout intervals [15]. The PSCSA use has most often been studied with propofol administration. There are many studies from the late 1990's to present trials concluding that PSCSA administration is both equivalent to physician conducted conventional sedation, and safe and effective in dressing changes of burn injuries, lithotripsy, endoscopic and radiological procedure [2][11].

Study

The first change of dressings after skin grafting in burn patients

Twenty patients were asked to participate in a study using a PSCSA to control pain and discomfort for their first dressing change after a skin grafting. Patients were provided by a single bolus of morphine IV 15 min before the procedure. The first 10 patients used a fixed bolus of propofol 0.3 mg/kg with a 5 min lockout. In the first 10 patients, there were no respiratory rates <10 breaths/min, systolic and diastolic blood pressure were

> within 25% of baseline values, and peripheral saturation stayed more than 94% with additional small flow oxygen via nasal cannual. The second group of 10, had a different PSCSA setup. The 2nd groups setup included an individualized propofol bolus, titrated to achieve a significant decrease of BIS or a sleepy state, and had no lockout period. The results showed the first group had double the demands than actual deliveries of propofol boluses. The second group of patients showed a more effective sedation, with respiratory and hemodynamic variables being not significantly different from the first group of patients [2].

Computer Assisted Personalized Sedation (CAPS)

The computer-assisted personalized sedation (CAPS) system is computerized system designed to help physician-nurse teams in the delivery of minimal to moderate propofol sedation to patients during procedures without anesthesia services. The CAPS system continually monitors and records in real time pulse oximetry, ECG, capnography, non-invasive blood pressure and patient responsiveness. The attractable features of this computerized system is that while continuously monitoring it detects early signs of potentially adverse physiology and level of sedation. This alert allows a physician-nurse team to adjust the infusion rate to an appropriate rate. It is also designed to react to signs of over-sedation by stopping or reducing delivery of propofol, increasing oxygen delivery and can even instruct the patient to deep breath [7].

Based on several studies the CAPS system was submitted to the U.S. FDA for premarket approval under the brand name, SEDASYS™ System. The Anesthesiology and Respiratory Therapy Devices Advisory Committee of the FDA voted 8 to 2 in favor of authorization of the SEDASYS™ System in May of 2009. On May 3rd 2013 the U.S. Food and Drug Administration (FDA) granted premarket approval (PMA) for the SEDASYS® System, the first computer-assisted personalized sedation (CAPS) system. The SEDASYS System has been granted for the intravenous administration of 1% (10 mg/mL) propofol injectable emulsion for the initiation and maintenance of minimal-to-moderate sedation, as defined by the American Society of Anesthesiologists (ASA) Continuum of Depth of Sedation. SEDAYS has been approved for the use in patients with an ASA physical status I and II, 18 years of age and older and for undergoing colonoscopy and esophagogastroduodenoscopy (EGD) procedures. The SEDASYS System is expected to be introduced on a limited basis beginning in 2014 to conduct two post-approval studies, which will monitor the use of the technology in actual clinical practice [6].

Target Controlled Infusion (TCI)

Another evolving technology currently used in Europe but not yet available in the United States, is target-controlled infusion (TCI). TCI has been developed as an standardized infusion delivery system which administers and achieves specific predicted target blood concentrations of opioids, propofol and other anesthetics. This delivery system administers IV agents via an infusion pump programmed to calculate and maintain the necessary infusion rate based on the pharmacokinetic model of a specific drug. Current TCI systems are known as open-loop or closed loop systems. Open loops operate using only a computer prediction of expected plasma concentration based on the drug profile and do not provide real time feedback. Closed loops on the other hand are a refinement of the TCI system which incorporates feedback from real time measures of sedation such as muscle relaxation. The advantage of the this refined system over the open loop system is that it is able to provide a more precise level of sedation with the administration of a lower concentration of drug [7][13].

It is not know if and when TCI will be available but what is know is that technology and the advancement of newer agents for the administration of sedation by non-anesthesiologist providers is on the rise. With the changes in healthcare reform for better quality and affordable care, and with the upcoming shortage of anesthesia providers, it reliable to say that the profession of a procedural sedation nurse will flourish. It may also be trustworthy to say that the procedural sedation nurse may also become a specialized field/profession much like a CRNA or anesthesia assistant.

Reference:

1. Brown, T. (2012, march 20). Anesthesia services used unnecessarily for gi endoscopies. *Medscape medial news*. Retrieved from http://www.medscape.com/viewarticle/760568

2. Chen, S., & Rex, D. (2004). registered nurse-administered propofol sedation for endoscopy. *Aliment Pharmacol Ther*, *19*(2), 147-55.

3. Coimbra, C., Choinière, M., & Hemmerling, T. (2003). Patient-controlled sedation using propofol for dressing changes in burn patients: A dose-finding study. *A&A*, *97*(3), 839-842.

4. Daugherty L, Fonseca R, Kumar KB, and Michaud P-C, An Analysis of the Labor Markets for Anesthesiology, Santa Monica, Calif: AND Corporation, TR-688-EES, 2010

5. Demiraran, Y., Korkut, E., Tamer, A., Yorulmaz, I., Kocaman, B., Sezen, G., & Akcan, Y. (2007). The comparison of dexmedetomidine and midazolam used for sedation of patients during upper endoscopy: A prospective, randomized study. *Can J Gastroenterol*, *21*(1), 25-29.

6. Division of Ethicon Endo-Surgery, Inc. (n.d.). Fda grants premarket approval (pma) for the sedasys® system for healthy patients undergoing sedation during routine colonoscopy and egd procedures. *PR News Wire*.

7. Guarracino, F., Lapolla, F., Cariello, C., Danella, A., Doroni, L., Baldassarri, R., Boldrini, A., & Volpe, M. (2005). Target controlled infusion: Tci. *Minerva anestesiologica*, *71*(6), 335-7. doi: DOI:10.1007/s00101-008-1332-z

8. the health care group. (2006). *facing the anesthesia shortage head-on: Crisis or opportunity*. Retrieved from www.healthcaregroup.com

9. Kost, M. (2004). Moderate sedation/analgesia. (2nd ed.). St. Louis: Saunders.

10. Lazear, S. E. (2011). Moderate sedation/analgesia. Sacremento, California: CME Resource. Retrieved from http://www.netce.com/courseoverview.php?courseid=751

11. Mazanikov, M., & Pöyhiä, R. (2011). Patient controlled sedation. *Duodecim*, *127*(9), 883-9.

12. *The shadow history of anesthesia.* (n.d.). Retrieved from http://science.howstuffworks.com/anesthesia6.htm

13. SGNA. (n.d.). *Sedation news*. Retrieved from http://www.sgna.org/Issues/SedationFactsorg/Resources_Updates/SedationNews.aspx

14. Smith PR. The cost of administering intravenous conscious sedation. Crit Care Nurs Cln North Am. 1997;9(3):423-427

15. Urman, R. D, & Kaye, A. D. (2012). Moderate and deep sedation in clinical practice. New York: Cambridge University Press.

Appendix

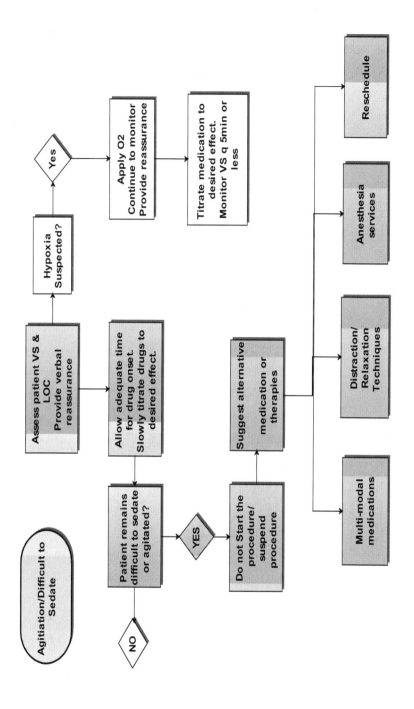

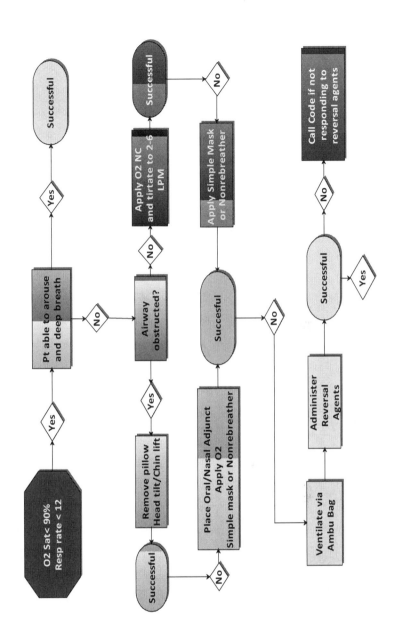

Oxygen Delivery Devices

Nasal Cannula
1-6LPM = 24-44% concentration of O2
FIO2 is increased by 4% per each LPM

Simple Face Mask
8-10LPM = 40-60% concentration of O2
O2 flow rate must be >5LPM to prevent CO_2 rebreathing

Non-Rebreather
6LPM = 60% concentration of O2
10LPM = 100% concentration of O2

Bag Valve Mask
Used for high delivery FIO2 and Ventilation

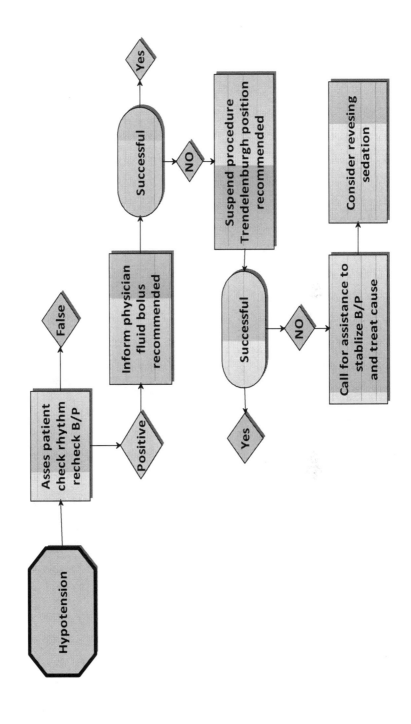

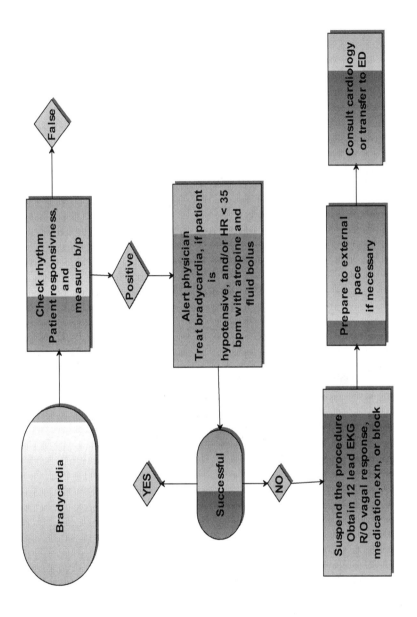

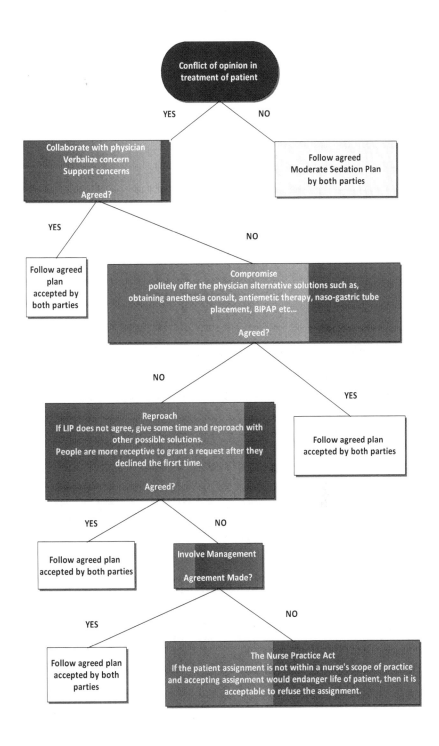

Paralytics (Neuromuscular Blockade Agents)

Paralytics (Neuromuscular Blockade Agents)			
Medication	Indication	Bolus Dose	Duration (Min)
Vecuronium		0.08-0.1mg/kg	25-30
Rocuronium		0.6-1.0mg/kg	30
Cisatracurium		0.1-0.2mg/kg	25
Succinylcholine	Rapid Sequence Intubation	1mg/kg	10

Organizations

- American Academy of Pediatrics (AAP)
- American Association of Nurse anesthetists (AANA)
- American College of Cardiology (ACC),
- American College of Emergency Physicians (ACEP)
- American College of Radiology (ACR)
- Society of Interventional Radiology (SIR)
- Association for Radiologic & Imaging Nursing (ARIN)
- American Association of Moderate Sedation Nurses (AAMSN) *
- American Society for Gastrointestinal Endoscopy (ASGE) *
- American Society of Anesthesiologists (ASA) *
- Association of PeriOperative Registered Nurses (AORN)
- University Health-System Consortium (UHC)

STOP BANG Questionnaire

Height _____ inches/cm Weight _____ lb/kg Age _____ Male/Female
BMI _____
Collar size of shirt: S, M, L, XL, or _____ inches/cm
Neck circumference* _____ cm

1. Snoring
Do you snore loudly (louder than talking or loud enough to be heard through closed doors)?
Yes No

2. Tired
Do you often feel tired, fatigued, or sleepy during daytime?
Yes No

3. Observed
Has anyone observed you stop breathing during your sleep?
Yes No

4. Blood pressure
Do you have or are you being treated for high blood pressure?
Yes No

5. BMI
BMI more than 35 kg/m2?
Yes No

6. Age
Age over 50 yr old?
Yes No

7. Neck circumference
Neck circumference greater than 40 cm?
Yes No

8. Gender
Gender male?
Yes No

* Neck circumference is measured by staff

High risk of OSA: answering yes to three or more items
Low risk of OSA: answering yes to less than three items

Reference Source: A Tool to Screen Patients for Obstructive Sleep Apnea, Frances Chung, F.R.C.P.C.,* Balaji Yegneswaran, M.B.B.S.,† Pu Liao, M.D.,‡ Sharon A. Chung, Ph.D.,§ Santhira Vairavanathan, M.B.B.S.,_ Sazzadul Islam, M.Sc.,_ Ali Khajehdehi, M.D.,† Colin M. Shapiro, F.R.C.P.C.#
Anesthesiology 2008; 108:812–21 Copyright © 2008, the American Society of Anesthesiologists, Inc. Lippincott Williams & Wilkins, Inc.

THE AUTHOR

A.G. Davis, a coal miner's daughter, was born and raised in West Virginia. At the age of seventeen, She volunteered her services in the United States Army, where she first started her journey in healthcare. The U.S Army trained her to be a practical nurse and an emergency medical technician. At age nineteen A.G. Davis began her nursing career working night shifts in a geriatric skilled facility, while pursing her associates degree. After working as a trauma, cardiac intensive care, home health and interventional radiology nurse, she continued to advance in her education. In 2009 Ms. Davis received her bachelor's in nursing. She has since demonstrated her commitment by providing and promoting optimal safe healthcare in the specialty of moderate sedation, endovascular stroke therapy, and interventional radiology specialties. She is a proud mountaineer that continues to strive for clinical, operational, and service excellence by encouraging commitment to high quality by focusing on improving the quality of nursing care delivery through education and mentorship. The basic tenets of her philosophy compel her at all levels to embrace a belief that nurses can always improve the quality of care they deliver.

Made in the USA
San Bernardino, CA
03 June 2016